Longevity Training-Book 8-Physical Body Health

This book is a transcription and reproduction of the training course materials from Course #8 "Physical Body Health"

Physical Body Health is the longest course in this Longevity training program.

It consists of three sections:

A) Supplements and Herbs for Longevity
B) Diets and Lifestyles of Long Lived People
C) Longevity related Weight and Exercise

These three areas are some of the most important aspects of caring for your Physical Body to improve your longevity.

Longevity Training-Book 8-Physical Body Health

Longevity Training-Book 8-Physical Body Health

Copyright Page

The book is copyrighted for 2018

Longevity Training-Book 8-Physical Body Health

By Martin K. Ettington

ISBN: 9781792078408

Printed in the United States of America

Longevity Training-Book 8-Physical Body Health

Longevity Training-Book 8-Physical Body Health

Other books by Martin K. Ettington

<u>Spiritual and Metaphysics Books:</u>
Prophecy: A History and How to Guide
God Like Powers and Abilities
Enlightenment for Newbies
Removing Illusions to Find True
    Happiness
Using the Scientific Method to Study
    the Paranormal
A Compendium of Metaphysics and
    How to Guides (Six books
    together in one volume)
Love from the Heart
The Enlightenment Experience
Learn Your Soul's Purpose
Pursuing Enlightenment
A Modern Man's Search for Truth
Use Intuition and Prophecy to Improve
    Your Life
The Handbook of Spiritual and Energy
    Healing

<u>Longevity & Immortality:</u>
Physical Immortality: A History and
    How to Guide
The Commentaries of Living Immortals
Records of Extremely Long Lived
    Persons
Enlightenment and Immortality
Longevity Improvements from Science
The 10 Principles of Personal
    Longevity
Telomeres & Longevity
The Diets and Lifestyles of the Worlds
    Oldest Peoples
The Longevity Six Books Bundle

<u>Science Fiction:</u>
Out of This Universe
Personal Freedom-Parts 1 & 2
The Psychic Soldier Series:
    Book 1-Himalayan Journey
    Book 2-A Soldier is Born
    Book 3-Fighting For Right
    Book 4-Earth Protector
The Immortality Sci Fi Bundle

<u>The God Like Powers Series:</u>
Human Invisibility
Invulnerability and Shielding
Teleportation
Psychokinesis
Our Energy Body, Auras, and
Thoughtforms

The God Like Powers Series—
    Volume 1 Compilation
<u>The Yoga Discovery Series:</u>
Yoga-An Ancient Art Form
Hatha Yoga-Helping you Live Better
Raja Yoga-Through the Ages
The Yoga Discovery Package

<u>Business & Coaching Books:</u>
Creating, Paublishing, & Marketing
    Practitioner Ebooks
Building a Successful Longevity
    Coaching Business
Why Become a Coach?
The Professional Coaching Success
Trilogy
2020-Make Money Writing and Selling
    Books
The 2020 Handbook of High Paying
    Work Without a College Degree

<u>Science, Technology, and Misc.</u>
Future Predictions By and Engineer &
    Seer
The Unusual Science & Technology
    Bundle
The Real Atlantis-In the Eye of the
    Sahara
Are Cryptozoological Animals Real or
    Imaginary?
Real Time Travel Stories From a
    Psychic Engineer
Removing Limits On Our
    Consciousness-And
    Thinking Outside the Box
33 Incredible True Survival Stories
How to Survive Anything: From the
    Wilderness to Man Made
    Disasters
All About Mars Journeys and
    Settlement
Mining the Asteroid Belt

<u>Ancient History</u>
The Real Atlantis-In the Eye of the
Sahara
Ancient & Prehistoric Civilizations
Ancient & Prehistoric Civilizations-Book
    Two
The History of Antediluvian Giants
The Antediluvian History of Earth
Ancient Underground Cities and
    Tunnels
Strange Objects Which Should Not Exist

Longevity Training-Book 8-Physical Body Health

Strange and Ancient Places in the USA
A Theory of Ancient Prehistory And
      Giant Aliens
<u>Aliens and Space</u>
Aliens and Secret Technology
Aliens Are Already Among Us
Designing and Building Space Colonies
Humanity and the Universe

All About Moon Bases
All About Mars Journeys and Settlement
The Space and Aliens Six Books Bundle
A Theory of Ancient Prehistory and
      Giant Aliens
The Space Colonies and Space
      Structures Coloring Book
All About Asteroids

<u>The Longevity Training Series</u>

(A transcription of the online Multimedia Longevity Coaching Training Program)

The Personal Longevity Training Series-Book1-Long Lived Persons
The Personal Longevity Training Series-Book2-Your Soul's Purpose
The Personal Longevity Training Series-Book3-Enable Your Life Urge
The Personal Longevity Training Series-Book4-Your Spiritual Connection
The Personal Longevity Training Series-Book5-Having Love in Your Heart
The Personal Longevity Training Series-Book6-Energy Body Health
The Personal Longevity Training Series-Book7-The Science of Longevity
The Personal Longevity Training Series-Book8-Physical Body Health
The Personal Longevity Training Series-Book9-Avoiding Accidents
The Personal Longevity Training Series-Book10-Implementing These Principles

The Personal Longevity Training Series-Books One Thru Ten

These books are all available in digital and printed formats from my
website and on Amazon, Barnes & Noble, Apple ITunes, and many other sites

My Books Website is: http://mkettingtonbooks.com

Longevity Training-Book 8-Physical Body Health

<u>Signup for our Mailing List to get the following:</u>

1) A discount coupon for 25% discount on all books on our site

2) Occasional Notices of new books available

3) Occasional Email on other offerings of ours (Monthly)

Go to this link to sign-up:

http://personal-longevity.com/mkebooks/emailsignup/

And click this link to get the FREE 102 page Ebook titled "Secrets of Many Things"

If you have any questions about this book or other subjects please contact the Author at:

mke@mkettingtonbooks.com

Longevity Training-Book 8-Physical Body Health

Table of Contents

Introduction

Back in 2008 I became very interested in the field of Longevity and Physical Immortality. After a lot of research this led me to my first book on the subject "Physical Immortality: A History and How to Guide". This book was pretty popular and I wanted to continue learning about Longevity and what things we could do about it in our lives.

The subject continued to fascinate me to the point that I developed a Longevity Coaching program over a couple of years starting in 2011. This online training program was multimedia—consisting of videos, my writings on longevity to read, online exercises, and tests for each of ten courses. It also included a lot of additional resources for each course including extra courses on how to become a successful Longevity Coach. A student who completed the training and tests successfully would become certified as a "Longevity Coach" and authorized to teach this material to others.

I developed a set of ten principles on longevity which are as follows:

The 10 Principles of Personal Longevity are:

- The Reality of Long Lived People
- Defining Your Purpose in Life
- Enabling the Life Urge
- Your Spiritual Health
- Having Love in Your Heart
- Energy Body Health
- The Science of Longevity
- Physical Body Health
- Using your Intuition for Safety
- Implementation of these principles

What are the 10 Principles all about?

The Reality of Long Lived People

The first principle is where I provide lots of evidence of people who have lived well over the age of 120 years old to 150-180-200, and even a 256 year old man from China:

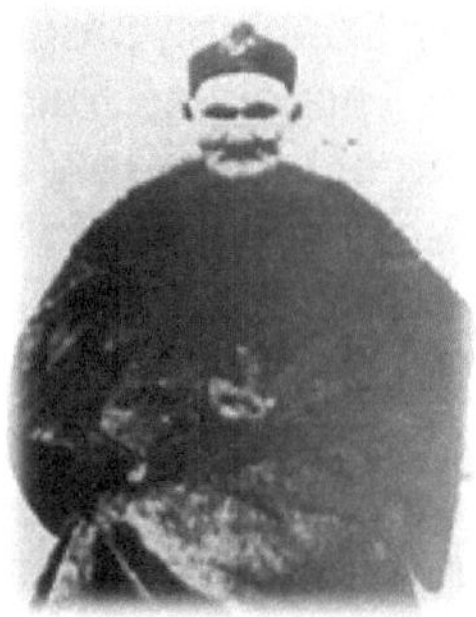

LI CHING-YUN: The Longest Lived person of record-256 Years (Source-The New York Times-May 6, 1933)

The Second Principle of Life Purpose

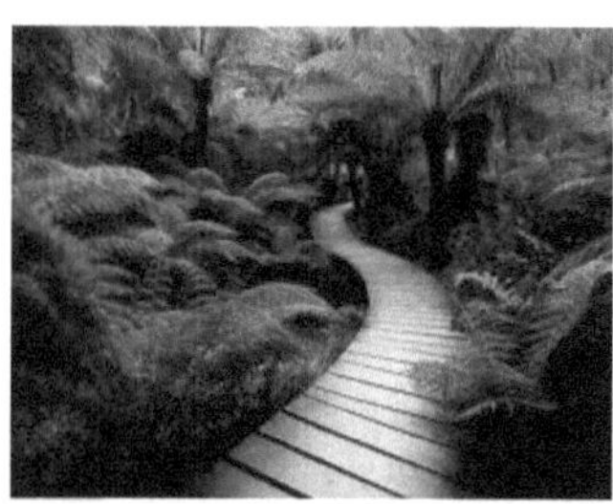

One of the things that occurred to me when I was putting the 10 principles together was that if one doesn't have a reason to live, or purpose in life--then what is the point?

This meant I had to add a very important step of how you can develop your own life purpose, or bring it up to date with your phase in life. Without reviewing your purpose-- then none of the rest of the principles matter.

Enabling the Life Urge

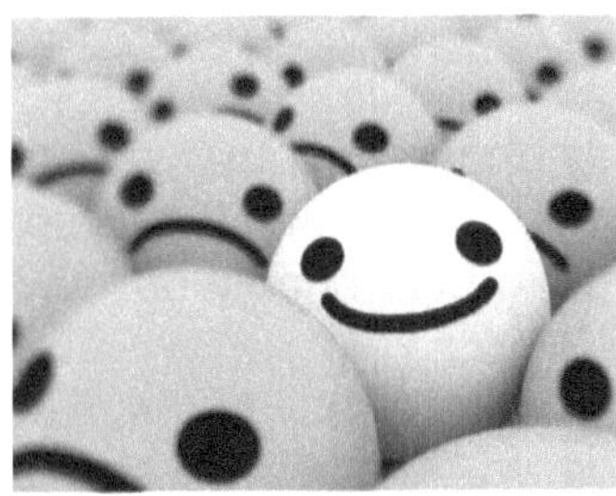

Have you ever realized how we are all programmed to expect to live through certain stages in life and then die? It's so common in our society that we don't think it odd that we expect to die at a certain age?

Have you ever heard radio ads saying "You are getting up in your sixties and seventies" so it's time to come out to our cemetery and buy a plot"

How ridiculous is this? And do you see how much our subconscious has been programmed towards death?

This principle is all about reprogramming ourselves to have a more positive outlook on life and its possibilities.

Having a Spiritual Connection in Your Life

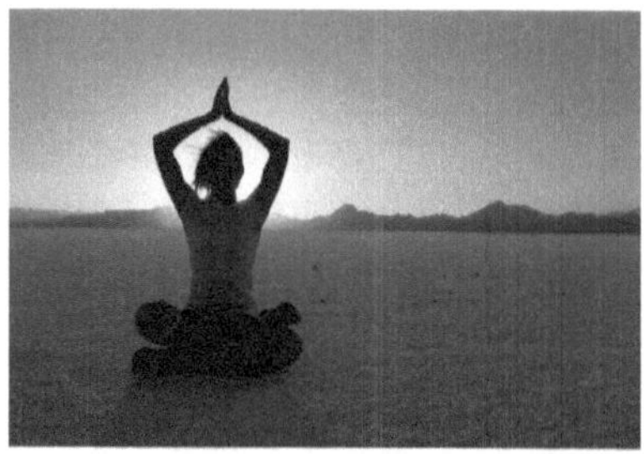

Most of us innately understand that we have a spiritual core in the center of our being. It is this spiritual core that we need to connect with to enable our physical health too.

It doesn't matter what religion you are. Regular meditation, deep prayer, or just walking in the woods helps you make and keep that connection in your life.

Having Love in Your Heart

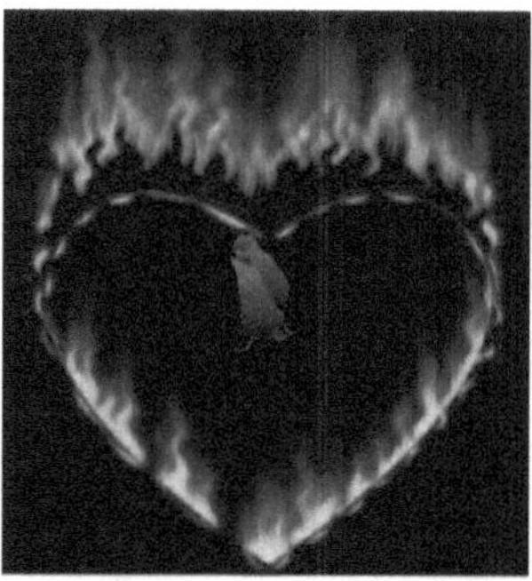

One of the most important things I learned in the last five years was that Unconditional Love is a real and physical thing. It is a powerful energy force in life and not just a philosophical belief system.

I considered it so important that I added it as a separate principle of longevity.

True Unconditional Love is healing, embodies happiness, and is a powerful part of our vital forces.

Energy Body Health

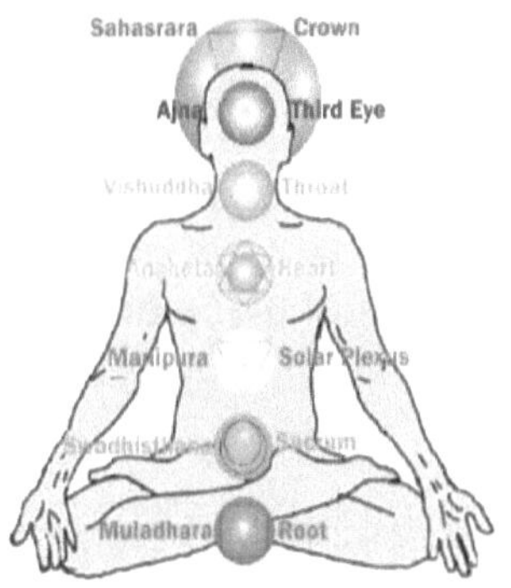

We all have an energy body which is part of our vital forces. The Indians talk about the "Chakras" and the Chinese talk about "Energy Meridians" in Acupuncture.

We should all learn different practices to keep our vital forces flowing for maximum health and vitality.

The Science of Longevity

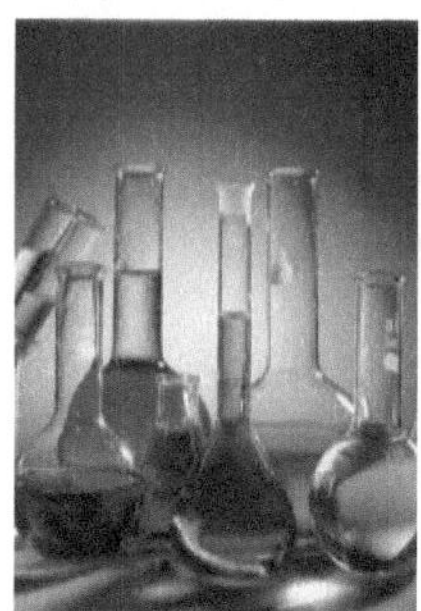

Science and Medicine are making new discoveries all the time that we can take advantage of to extend our lives. Why not take advantage of these discoveries which provide new therapies and supplements to increase our longevity.

There is also a lot we can learn from plants and animals. We all share the same genetic basis.

Some of these plants and animals live thousands of years and some cells are immortal.

What can we learn from them to apply to our lives?

Physical Body Health

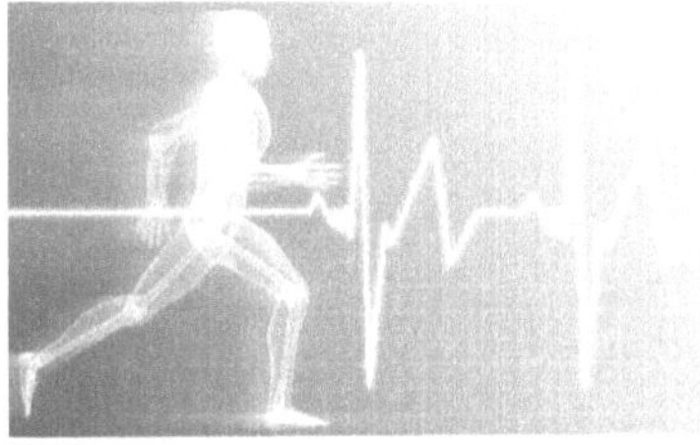

There are many types of supplements used for anti-aging for thousands of years. What can we learn about them that we can apply to our lives?

What other considerations about our physical health does nontraditional or alternative medicine offer?

Using Your Intuition for Safety

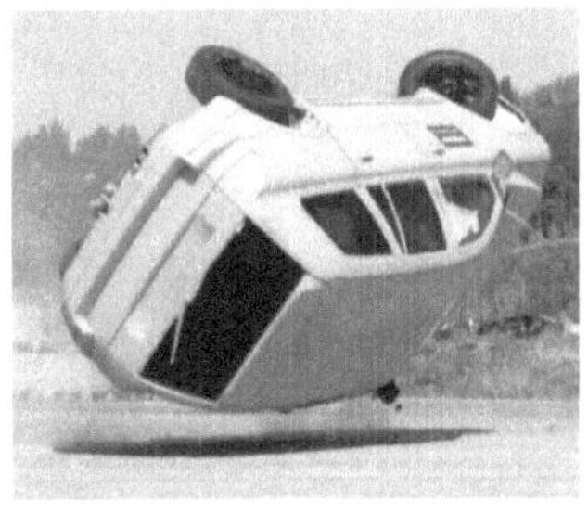

Once you have established your own long term health then what is the greatest danger you face?

ACCIDENTS

We can learn to use our intuition to make us safer as well as see potential future events which may be good too.

Why not open up to the possibilities of how our spirit has this natural ability in all of us?

Implementing These Principles in Your Life

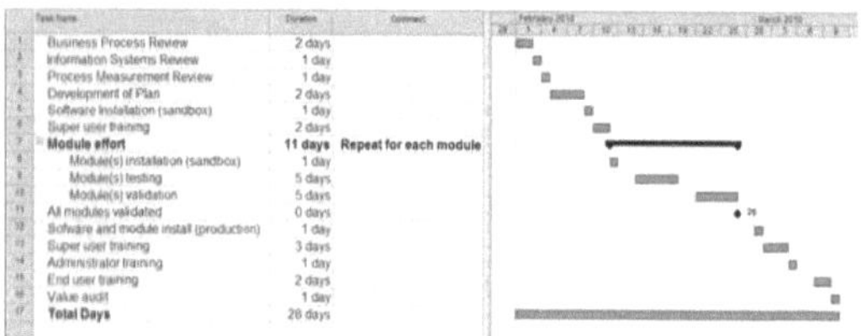

It's nice to read about all these concepts, but how can you really apply them to your own life?

This is what the chapter on implementation is all about, and it helps you plan a lifelong change in your health focus to live these principles and truly experience long term health, greater happiness, and extended longevity.

For five years I amended and improved these materials which now include a lot more information and helpful concepts for students wanting to improve their longevity and those of others.

I transcribed my videos and other materials to this book so you can read it all, and later hear it in an AudioBook.

This book is priced pretty inexpensively, compared to the online training and certification program which sells in total for $1,995 USD. If you are interested in taking the entire online program at a major discount, then please contact me at:

Marty@personal-longevity.com

Hope you enjoy these materials since when applied correctly they will significantly change your life.

PLP Concepts Overview

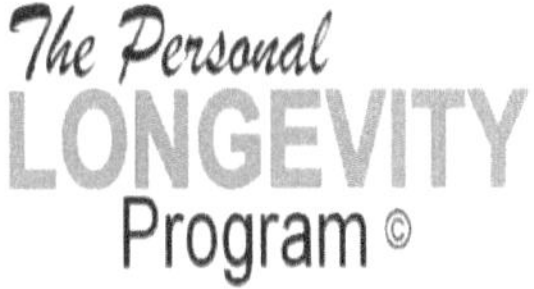

(Transcription of overview video)

Hello I'm Martin Ettington and I'd like to introduce you to the Personal Longevity Program which is an integrated holistic approach to long-term health. In this video we will only cover the high level concepts which comprise individual courses in the coaching certificate program for personal longevity.

The first concept is that long lived people exist and have existed for hundreds of thousands of years. We cover in the first course all about their records; along with people not only in places you might think like India, but in Europe and the United States-people who've lived long lives and well documented cases.

We discuss people who have lived well over the age of 120 and even the case of a Chinaman who lived to 256 years old. Plus a lot of mythology about people who have lived even longer lives so you get an idea that extending your life much longer than we think is currently medically and scientifically possible is certainly something that can happen.

The second course's concept has to do with finding your souls purpose. The point of wanting to live a long life is to know what your purpose in life is, so we go through some readings and some exercises to help you determine where soul's purpose in life is. Then doing goals as a fundamental concept so you will know the motivations in your life.

Third is the "Psychology of Living" also known by certain practitioners as "Removing the death Urge". The psychology of living has to do with seeking a positive image about your ability to live a long time. We tend to be programmed from birth about the idea that we are going to go through certain stages in our life as a child, as a teenager, and as adults. It's about reprogramming your subconscious as to the possibilities of a long life.

I've also learned in my life that it is very important to be able open your heart to unconditional love. When you're able to love unconditionally it also helps increase the strength of your immune system and fight off disease. So this is an aspect of spiritual growth. The courses also cover unconditional love and energy body forces. Managing your energy body is an important component of who you are in having energy working properly in your body and is another aspect of health for the length of longevity.

There are many types of scientific and medical research which are being done today and which will contribute to human longevity in the future.

Do you know that the average lifespan in the United States in 1900 was only about 40 years? We have doubled lifespan in the last century with current technologies but things under way in terms of scientific and medical improvements will help extend your lives further.

Also in this course on longevity we will cover a lot of the concepts which are being researched by scientists today. There are suggestions for more things you can do to do to use this science to improve your health along with physical supplements.

A unique thing that I thought about and decided to offer in these courses has to do with all my experiences in prophecy and how I was able to change outcomes on accidents that would occur to me by using simple exercises you can learn to change these outcomes. If you're in great health often the biggest thing you have to worry about are accidents.

We also provide guidelines you can follow on a daily basis and plans you can make to live healthier and happier and have a much longer life than you ever thought possible.

Thank you for listening !

Course #8A Intro Video

(Transcription of Video)

Hello this is Marty Ettington. I'd like to welcome you to course number eight on the "Physical Body Health" as part of the personal longevity program. The personal longevity program philosophy is designed to be an encompassing holistic approach built on top of current medical and scientific health practices.

There's millions of pages of science and medical information about taking care of your physical body which I'm not going to try and repeat here in this course. We're going to focus on some alternative medicine and supplement options which are known to be able to enhance your long-term health.

Many people swear by longevity supplements that they take. The categories of approaches which are included are several different books on natural remedies and cures and also I thought it was important to learn something about Chinese herbalism which is the basis for many longevity supplements and treatments. And some of these supplements which can prolong your life. Or ones for instance like the guy who was two hundred fifty six years old who spent a hundred years as an herbalist. As Ginseng tea and then there's a series of articles on other longevity supplements with a lot of recommendations. You'll have some assignments on that. Healthy yoga and other physical practices are lots of things to help increase your information about natural cures herbalism and practices you can do for your physical body so I hope you enjoy this course. Thank You very much

8A-Physical Body Health—Supplements-From Nature's Cures

(Natural Healing –Extracts from Nature's Cures)

Principles and Practice of Nature Cure

Nature Cures, not the Physician. – Hippocrates

Nature cure is a constructive method of treatment which aims at removing the basic cause of disease through the rational use of the elements freely available in nature. It is not only a system of healing, but also a way of life, in tune with the internal vital forces or natural elements comprising the human body. It is a complete revolution in the art and science of living.

Although the term 'naturopathy' is of relatively recent origin, the philosophical basis and several of the methods of nature cure treatments are ancient. It was practiced in ancient Egypt, Greece and Rome. Hippocrates, the father of medicine (460-357 B.C.) strongly advocated it. India, it appears, was much further advanced in older days in natural healing system than other countries of the world. There are references in India's ancient sacred books about the extensive use of nature's excellent healing agents such as air, earth, water and sun. The Great Baths of the Indus Valley civilization as discovered at Mohenjo-Daro in old Sind testifies to the use of water for curative purposes in ancient India.

The modern methods of nature cure originated in Germany in 1822, when Vincent Priessnitz established the first hydropathic establishment there. With his great success in water cure, the idea of drugless healing spread throughout the civilized world and many medical practitioners throughout the civilized world and many medical practitioners from America and other countries became his enthusiastic students and disciples. These students subsequently enlarged and developed the various methods of natural healing in their own way. The whole mass of knowledge was later collected under one name, Naturopathy. The credit for the name Naturopathy goes to Dr. Benedict Lust (1872 - 1945), and hence he is called the Father of Naturopathy.

Nature cure is based on the realization that man is born healthy and strong and that he can stay as such as living in accordance with the laws of nature. Even if born with some inherited affliction, the individual can eliminate it by putting to the best use the natural agents of healing. Fresh air, sunshine, a proper diet, exercise, scientific relaxation, constructive thinking and the right mental attitude, along with prayer and meditation all play their part in keeping a sound mind in a sound body.

Nature cure believes that disease is an abnormal condition of the body resulting from the violation of the natural laws. Every such violation has repercussions on the human system in the shape of lowered vitality, irregularities of the blood and lymph and the accumulation of waste matter and toxins. Thus, through a faulty diet it is not the digestive system alone which is adversely affected. When toxins accumulate, other organs such as the bowels, kidneys, skin and lungs are overworked and cannot get rid of these harmful substances as quickly as they are produced.

Besides this, mental and emotional disturbances cause imbalances of the vital electric field within which cell metabolism takes place, producing toxins. When the soil of this electric field is undisturbed, disease-causing germs can live in it without multiplying or producing toxins. It is only when it is disturbed or when the blood is polluted with toxic waste that the germs multiply and become harmful.

Basic Principles

The whole philosophy and practice of nature cure is built on three basic principles. These principles are based on the conclusions reached from over a century of effective naturopathic treatment of diseases in Germany, America and Great Britain. They have been tested and proved over and over again by the results obtained.

The first and most basic principle of nature cure is that all forms of disease are due to the same cause, namely, the accumulations of waste materials and bodily refuse in the system. These waste materials in the healthy individual are removed from the system through the organs of elimination. But in the diseased person, they are steadily piling up in the body through years of faulty habits of living such as wrong feeding, improper care of the body and habits contributing to enervation and nervous exhaustion such as worry, overwork and excesses of all kinds. It follows from this basic principle that the only way to cure disease is to employ methods which will enable the system to throw off these toxic accumulations. All natural treatments are actually directed towards this end.

The second basic principle of nature cure is that all acute diseases such as fevers, colds, inflammations, digestive disturbances and skin eruptions are nothing more than self-initiated efforts on the part of the body to throw off the accumulated waste materials and that all chronic diseases such as heart disease, diabetes, rheumatism, asthma, kidney disorders, are the results of continued suppression of the acute diseases through harmful methods such as drugs, vaccines, narcotics and gland extracts.

The third principle of nature cure is that the body contains an elaborate healing mechanism which has the power to bring about a return to normal condition of health, provided right methods are employed to enable it to do so. In other words, the power to cure disease lies within the body itself and not in the hands of the doctor.

Nature Cure vs Modern System

The modern medical system treats the symptoms and suppresses the disease but does little to ascertain the real cause. Toxic drugs which may suppress or relieve some ailments usually have harmful side-effects. Drugs usually hinder the self-healing efforts of the body and make recovery more difficult. According to the late Sir William Osler, an eminent physician and surgeon, when drugs are used, the patient has to recover twice - once from the illness, and once from the drug. Drugs cannot cure diseases; disease continues. It is only its pattern that changes. Drugs also produce dietary deficiencies by destroying nutrients, using them up, and preventing their absorption. Moreover, the toxicity they produce occurs at a time when the body is least capable of coping with it. The power to restore health thus lies not in drugs, but in nature. The approach of modern system is more on combative lines after the disease has set in, whereas nature cure system lays greater emphasis on preventive method and adopts measures to attain and maintain health and prevent disease. The modern medical system treats each disease as a separate entity, requiring specific drug for its cure, whereas the nature cure system treats the organism as a whole and seeks to restore harmony to the whole of the patient's being.

Methods of Nature Cure

The nature cure system aims at the readjustment of the human system from abnormal to normal conditions and functions, and adopts methods of cure which are in conformity with the constructive principles of nature. Such methods remove from the system the accumulation of toxic matter and poisons without in any way injuring the vital organs of the body. They also stimulate the organs of elimination and purification to better functioning.

To cure disease, the first and foremost requirement is to regulate the diet. To get rid of accumulated toxins and restore the equilibrium of the system, it is desirable to completely exclude acid-forming foods, including proteins, starches and fats, for a week or more and to confine the diet to fresh fruits which will disinfect the stomach and alimentary canal. If the body is overloaded with morbid matter, as in acute disease, a complete fast for a few days may be necessary for the elimination of toxins. Fruit juice may, however, be taken during a fast. A simple rule is: do not eat when you are sick, stick to a light diet of fresh fruits. Wait for the return of the usual healthy appetite. Loss of appetite is Nature's warning that no burden should be placed on the digestive organs. Alkaline foods such as raw vegetables and sprouted whole grain cereals may be added after a week of a fruits-only diet. Another important factor in the cure of diseases by natural methods is to stimulate the vitality of the body. This can be achieved by using water in various ways and at varying temperatures in the form of packs or baths. The application of cold water, especially to the abdomen, the seat of most diseases, and to the sexual organs, through a cold sitting (hip) bath immediately lowers body heat and stimulates the nervous system. In the form of wet packs, hydrotherapy offers a simple natural method of abating fevers and reducing pain and inflammation without any harmful side-effects. Warm water applications, on the other hand, are relaxing. Other natural methods useful in the cure of diseases are air and sunbaths, exercise and massage.

 Air and sunbaths revive dead skin and help maintain it in a normal condition. Exercise, especially yogic asanas, promotes inner health and harmony and helps eliminate all tension : physical, mental and emotional. Massage tones up the nervous system and quickens blood circulation and the metabolic process. Thus a well-balanced diet, sufficient physical exercise, the observation of the other laws of well-being such as fresh air, plenty of sunlight, pure drinking water, scrupulous cleanliness, adequate rest and right mental attitude can ensure proper health and prevent disease.

Miracles of Alkalizing Diet

The human body is composed of various organs and parts, which are made up of tissues and cells. These tissues and cells are composed of 16 chemical elements. The balance or equilibrium of these chemical elements in the body is an essential factor in the maintenance of health and healing of disease. The acid-alkaline balance plays a vital role in this balanced body chemistry. All foods, after digestion and absorption leave either an acid or alkaline ash in the body depending on their mineral composition. The normal body chemistry is approximately 20 per cent acid and 80 per cent alkaline.

This is the acid-alkaline balance. In normal health, the reaction of the blood is alkaline and that is essential for our physical and mental well-being. The preponderance of alkalis in the blood is due to the fact that the products of the vital combustions taking place in the body are mostly acid in character. Carbohydrates and fats form about nine-tenths of the normal fuel of the body. In normal health, this great mass of material is converted into carbon dioxide gas and water. Half of the remaining one-tenth fuel is also converted into the same gas and water. This huge amount of acid is transported by the blood to the various points of discharge, mainly the lungs. By virtue of alkalinity, the blood is able to transport the acid from the tissues to the discharge points.

Acidosis

Whenever the alkalinity of the blood is reduced, even slightly, its ability to transport the carbon dioxide gets reduced. This results in the accumulation of acid in the tissues. This condition is known as acidosis or hypo-alkalinity of the blood. Its symptoms are hunger, indigestion, burning sensation and pain in the pharynx, nausea, vomiting, headache, various nervous disorders and drowsiness. Acidosis is the breeding ground for most diseases.

Nepthritis or Bright's disease, rheumatism, premature old age, arteriosclerosis, high blood pressure, skin disorders and various degenerative diseases are traceable to this condition. It seriously interferes with the functions of the glands and organs of the body. It also lowers the vitality of the system, thereby increasing the danger of infectious diseases. The main cause of acidosis or hypo-alkalinity of the blood is faulty diet, in which too many acid forming foods have been consumed. In the normal process of metabolism or converting the food into energy by the body, various acids are formed in the system and in addition, other acids are introduced in food. Whenever there is substantial increase in the formation of acids in the system and these acids are not properly eliminated through the lungs, the kidneys and the bowels, the alkalinity of the blood is reduced, resulting in acidosis. Other causes of acidosis are depletion of alkali reserve due to diarrhea, dysentery, cholera etc., accumulation of carbon dioxide in asphyxia and anoxia as in circulatory and pulmonary diseases and accumulation of acetone bodies resulting from starvation, vomiting and diabetes mellitus.

Acidosis can be prevented by maintaining a proper ratio between acid and alkaline foods in the diet. Certain foods leave alkaline ash and help in maintaining the alkalinity of the food, while others leave highly acid ash and lower the alkali reserve of the blood and tissue fluids to a very large extent. Eggs do the same but less strongly than meats. Cereals of all kinds, including all sorts of breads are also acid-forming foods, though much less than meats. All fruits, with exceptions like plums and prunes and all green and root vegetables are highly alkaline foods and help to alkalinize the blood and other tissue fluids. Thus, our daily diet should consist of four-fifth of alkaline-forming foods such as juicy fruits, tubers, legumes, ripe fruits, leafy and root vegetables and one fifty of acid-forming foods containing concentrated proteins and starches such as meat, fish, bread and cereals.

Eating sensibly in this manner will ensure the necessary alkalinity of the food which will keep the body in perfect health. Whenever a person has acidosis, the higher the ratio of alkaline forming foods in his diet, the quicker will be the recovery. Acids are neutralized by alkalies. It is, therefore, imperative that persons suffering from various ailments are given adequate alkaline ash foods to offset the effects of acid-forming foods and leave a safe margin of alkalinity. The most agreeable and convenient means of alkalizing the blood are citrus fruits and fruit juices. The alkalizing value of citrus fruits are due to large percentage of alkaline salts, mainly potash, which they contain. Each pint of orange juice contains 12 grains of potassium, one of the most potent of alkalis. Lemon juice contains nine grains of the alkali to the pint and grape seven grains.

Diet in Disease

In the diet during disease, breakfast may consist of fresh fruits, lunch may comprise raw vegetables with acid and sub-acid fruits, and for dinner raw and cooked vegetables, or light starchy vegetables like beet, carrot, cauliflower, egg-plant and squashes may be taken. Sweet fruits may be added to this diet after seven days. Foods are classified as acid-producing or alkaline-producing depending on their reaction on the urine. Calcium, magnesium, sodium and potassium present in foods contribute to the alkaline effect, while sulphur, phosphorous and chlorine contribute to the acidic effect.

Depending on the pre-dominating constituents in a particular food, it is classified as acid-forming or alkaline-forming. The effect of food stuffs upon the alkalinity of the blood depends upon their residue which they leave behind after undergoing oxidation in the body. It is an error to presume that because a food tastes acid, it has an acidic reaction in the blood. For instance, fruits and vegetables have organic acids in combination with soda and potash in the form of acid salts. When the acids are burnt or utilized in the body, the alkaline soda or potash is left behind. Hence the effect of the natural fruit acids is to increase the alkalinity of the blood rather than reduce it. Based on the above observations, the following charts show the common foods with acid and alkaline ash:

A - Foods Leaving An Acid Ash (One-Fifth Class)

Barley Eggs
Bananas (unripe)
Grain Foods
Beans Lentils
Bread Meats
Cereals Nuts except almonds
Cakes
Oatmeal
Chicken Peas
Confections
Rice
Corn Sugar
Chorolate Sea Foods
Coffee
Tea

B - Foods Leaving An Alkaline Ash (Four-fifths class)

Almonds
Melons
Apples
Milk
Apricots
Onions
Banana (ripe)
Oranges
Beets
Parsley
Cabbage
Peaches
Carrots
Pears
Cauliflower
Pineapple
Celery
Potatoes
Coconuts
Pumpkins
Cottage Cheese
Radishes
Cucumbers
Raisins
Dates
Spinach
Figs (Fresh and Dry)
Soybeans
Grapes
Tomatoes
Lemons
Turnips
Lettuce

Vitamins and their Importance in Health and Disease

Natures Cures-Chapter 12

The word 'Vitamin' meaning a vital amine was proposed by a Polish Researcher, Dr. Cacimir Funk, in 1911 to designate a new food substance which cured beri-beri.

Other terms were proposed as new factors were discovered. But the word vitamin, with the final 'e' dropped, met with popular favor. Vitamins are potent organic compounds which are found in small concentrations in foods.

They perform specific and vital functions in the body chemistry. They are like electric sparks which help to run human motors. Except for a few exceptions, they cannot be manufactured or synthesized by the organism and their absence or improper absorption results in specific deficiency disease. It is not possible to sustain life without all the essential vitamins. In their natural state they are found in minute quantities in organic foods. We must obtain them from these foods or in dietary supplements. Vitamins, which are of several kinds, differ from each other in physiological function, in chemical structure and in their distribution in food. They are broadly divided into two categories, namely, fat-soluble and water-soluble. Vitamins A, D, E and K are all soluble in fat and fat solvents and are therefore, known as fat-soluble. They are not easily lost by ordinary cooking methods and they can be stored in the body to some extent, mostly in the liver. They are measured in international units.

Vitamin B Complex and C are water soluble. They are dissolved easily in cooking water. A portion of these vitamins may actually be destroyed by heating. They cannot be stored in body and hence they have to be taken daily in foods. Any extra quantity taken in any one day is eliminated as waste. Their values are given in milligrams and micrograms, whichever is appropriate. Vitamins, used therapeutically, can be of immense help in fighting disease and speeding recovery.

They can be used in two ways, namely, correcting deficiencies and treating disease in place of drugs. Latest researches indicate that many vitamins taken in large doses far above the actual nutritional needs, can have a miraculous healing effect in a wide range of common complaints and illnesses. Vitamin therapy has a distinct advantage over drug therapy. While drugs are always toxic and have many undesirable side effects, vitamins, as a rule are non-toxic and safe. The various functions of common vitamins, their deficiency symptoms, natural sources, daily requirements and their therapeutic uses are discussed in brief as follows:

Vitamin A

Known as anti-opathalmic, vitamin A is essential for growth and vitality. It builds up resistance to respiratory and other infections and works mainly on the eyes, lungs, stomach and intestines. It prevents eye diseases and plays a vital role in nourishing the skin and hair. It helps to prevent premature ageing and senility, increases life expectancy and extends youthfulness. The main sources of this vitamin are fish liver oil, liver, whole milk, curds, pure ghee, butter, cheese, cream and egg yolk, green leafy and certain yellow root vegetables such as spinach, lettuce, turnip, beets, carrot, cabbage and tomato and ripe fruits such as prunes, mangoes, pappaya, apricots, peaches, almonds and other dry fruits.

A prolonged deficiency of vitamin A may result in inflammation of the eyes, poor vision, frequent colds, night blindness and increased susceptibility to infections, lack of appetite and vigor, defective teeth and gums and skin disorders.

The recommended daily allowance of vitamin A is 5,000 international units for adults and 2,600 to 4,000 international units for children. When taken in large therapeutic doses, which are usually 25,000 to 50,000 units a day, it is highly beneficial in the treatment of head and chest colds, sinus trouble, influenza and other infectious diseases. It is also valuable in curing night blindness and other eye diseases as well as many stubborn skin disorders. This vitamin can be given up to 100,000 units a day for a limited period of four weeks under doctor's supervision. In a recent year-long study, huge doses of vitamin A given twice a year reduced death by about Vitamins and their Importance in Health and Disease 30 per cent among Indonesian children. This has raised the hope in the fight against a significant cause of childhood mortality in developing countries.

B COMPLEX VITAMINS

There are a large variety of vitamins in the B group, the more important being B1 or thiamine, B2 or riboflavin, B3 or niacin or nicotinic acid, B6 or pyridoxine, B9 or folic acid, B12 and B5 or pantothenic acid. B vitamins are synergistic. They are more potent together than when used separately.

THIAMINE

Known as anti-beberi, anti-neuritic and anti-ageing vitamin, thiamine plays an important role in the normal functioning of the nervous system, the regulation of carbohydrates and good digestion. It protects heart muscle, stimulates brain action and helps prevent constipation. It has a mild diuretic effect. Valuable sources of this vitamin are wheat germ, yeast, the outer layer of whole grains, cereals, pulses, nuts, peas, legumes, dark green leafy vegetables, milk, egg, banana, and apple.

The deficiency of thiamine can cause serious impairment of the digestive system and chronic constipation, loss of weight, diabetes, mental depression, nervous exhaustion and weakness of the heart. The recommended daily allowance for this vitamin is about two milligrams for adults and 1.2 mg. for children. The need for this vitamin increases during illness, stress and surgery as well as during pregnancy and lactation. When taken in a large quantity, say up to 50 mg it is beneficial in the treatment of digestive disorders, neuritis and other nervous troubles as well as mental depression. For best results, all other vitamins of B group should be administered simultaneously. Prolonged ingestion of large doses of any one of the isolated B complex vitamins may result in high urinary losses of other B-vitamins and lead to deficiencies of these vitamins.

RIBOFLAVIN

Vitamin B2 or riboflavin, also known as vitamin G, is essential for growth and general health as also for healthy eyes, skin, nails and hair. It helps eliminate sore mouth, lips and tongue. It also functions with other substances to metabolize carbohydrates, fats, and protein. The main sources of this vitamin are green leafy vegetables, milk, cheese, wheat germ, egg, almonds, sunflower, seeds, citrus fruits and tomatoes. Its deficiency can cause a burning sensation in the legs, lips and tongue, oily skin, premature wrinkles on face and arm and eczema. The recommended daily allowance for this vitamin is 1.6 to 2.6 mg. for adults and 0.6 to one mg for children. Its use in larger quantities, say from 25 to 50 mg. is beneficial in the treatment of nutritional cataracts and other eye ailments, digestive disturbances, nervous depression, general debility, and certain types of high blood pressure.

NIACIN

Vitamin B3 or niacin or nicotinic acid is essential for proper circulation, healthy functioning of the nervous system and proper protein and carbohydrate metabolism. It is essential for synthesis of sex hormones, cartisone, thyroxin and insulin. It is contained in liver, fish, poultry, peanut, whole wheat, green leafy vegetables, dates, figs, prunes and tomato. A deficiency can lead to skin eruptions, frequent stools, mental depression, insomnia, chronic headaches, digestives disorders and anemia. The recommended daily allowance is 12 to 20 mg. for adults and 4.8 to 12 mg. for children. Large doses of this vitamin say up to 100 mg. with each meal, preferably together with other B group vitamins, affords relief in case of migraine and high blood pressure caused by nervousness, high cholesterol and arteriosclerosis.

PYRIDOXINE

Vitamin B6 or pyridoxine is actually a group of substances - pyridoxine, pyridoxinal and pyridoxamine - that are closely related and function together. It helps in the absorption of fats and proteins, prevents nervous and skin disorders and protects against degenerative diseases. The main sources of this vitamin are yeast, wheat, bran, wheat germ, pulses, cereals, banana, walnuts, soybeans, milk, egg, liver, meat and fresh vegetables. Deficiency can lead to dermatitis, conjunctivitis, anemia, depression, skin disorders, nervousness, insomnia, migraine Vitamins and their headaches and heart diseases. The recommended daily requirement is 2.0 mg. for adults and 0.2 mg. for children. This vitamin used therapeutically from 100 to 150 mg. daily can relieve painful joints and the discomforts of pregnancy and pre-menstrual symptoms. Vitamin B6 is now the most intensively studied of all vitamins.

Researches are on the threshold of a number of promising developments involving treatments of various ailments with this vitamin. They include hyperactivity in children, asthma, arthritis, kidney stones, blood clots in heart attack victims and nervous disorders.

FOLIC ACID

Vitamin B9 or folic acid, along with vitamin B12 is necessary for the formation of red blood cells. It is essential for the growth and division of all body cells for healing processes. It aids protein metabolism and helps prevent premature greying. Valuable sources of this vitamin are deep green leafy vegetables such as spinach, lettuce, brewers yeast, mushrooms, nuts, peanuts and liver. A deficiency can result in certain types of anemia, serious skin disorders, loss of hair, impaired circulation, fatigue and mental depression. The minimum daily requirement of this vitamin is 0.4 mg. To correct anemia and deficiencies 5 mg or more are needed daily. Some authorities believe that folic acid is contraindicated in leukemia and cancer.

PANTOTHENIC ACID

Vitamin B5 or pantothenic acid helps in cell building, maintaining normal growth and development of the central nervous system. It stimulates the adrenal glands and increases the production of cortisone and other adrenal hormones. It is essential for conversion of fatty and sugar to energy. It also helps guard against most physical and mental stresses and toxins and increases vitality. The main sources of this vitamin are whole grain bread and cereals, green vegetables, peas, beans, peanuts and egg yolk. It can be synthesized in the body by intestinal bacteria. A deficiency can cause chronic fatigue, hypoglycemia, greying and loss of hair, mental depression, stomach disorders, blood and skin disorders. The minimum daily requirement of this vitamin has not been established, but is estimated to be between 30 and 50 mg a day. The usual therapeutic doses are 50 to 200 mg. In some studies, 1,000 mg or more were given daily for six months without side effects. It is useful in the treatment of insomnia, low blood pressure and hypoglycemia or low blood sugar.

VITAMIN B12

Vitamin B12 or cobolamin, commonly known as "red vitamin", is the only vitamin that contains essential mineral elements. It is essential for proper functioning of the central nervous system, production and regeneration of red blood cells and proper utilization of fat, carbohydrates and protein for body building. It also improves concentration, memory and balance. Valuable sources of this vitamin are kidney, liver, meat, milk, eggs, bananas and peanuts. Its deficiency can lead to certain types of anemia, poor appetite and loss of energy and mental disorders. The recommended daily allowance of this vitamin is 3 mcg. Taken in large therapeutic doses from 50 to 100 mcg., it is beneficial in the treatment of lack of concentration, fatigue, depression, insomnia and poor memory.

VITAMIN C

Vitamin C or ascorbic acid is essential for normal growth and the maintenance of practically all the body tissues, especially those of the joints, bones, teeth, and gums. It protects one against infections and acts as a harmless antibiotic. It promotes healing and serves as protection against all forms of stress and harmful effects of toxic chemicals. It helps prevent and cure the common cold. It also helps in decreasing blood cholesterol. This vitamin is found in citrus fruits, berries, green and leafy vegetables, tomatoes, potatoes, sprouted bengal and green grams, A deficiency can cause scurvy marked by weakness, anemia, bleeding gums and painful and swollen parts, slow healing of sores and wounds, premature ageing and lowered resistance to all infections. The recommended daily allowance is 50 to 75 mg. for adults and 30 to 50 mg. for children. Smokers and older persons have greater need for vitamin C. It is used therapeutically in huge doses from 100 to 10,000mg. a day. It prevents and cures colds and infections effectively, neutralizes various toxins in the system, speeds healing processes in virtually all cases of ill health, increases sexual vitality and prevents premature ageing. According to Dr. Linus Pauling, a world famous chemist and nutrition expert, "because vitamin C is one of the least toxic vitamins, it is very safe to use in high doses. " Your body will take exactly what it needs and excrete any excess naturally."

VITAMIN D

Vitamin D is necessary for proper bone and teeth formation and for the healthy functioning of the thyroid gland. It assists in the assimilation of calcium, phosphorus and other minerals from the digestive tract. This vitamin is found in the rays of the sun, fish, milk, eggs, butter and sprouted seeds. A deficiency can cause gross deformation of bones and severe tooth decay. The recommended daily allowance of this vitamin for both adults and children is 400 to 500 international units. Therapeutically, up to 4,000 to 5,000 units a day for adult or half of this for children, is a safe dose, if taken for not longer than one month. It is beneficial in the treatment of muscular fatigue, constipation and nervousness. It can be toxic if taken in excessive doses, especially for children. Signs of toxicity are unusual thirst, sore eyes, itching skin, vomiting, diarrhea, urinary urgency, abnormal calcium deposits in blood vessel walls, liver, lungs, kidneys and stomach.

VITAMIN E

Vitamin E is essential for normal reproductory functions, fertility and physical vigor. It prevents unsaturated fatty acids, sex hormones and fat soluble vitamins from being destroyed in the body by oxygen. It dilutes blood vessels and improves circulation. It is essential for the prevention of heart diseases, asthma, arthritis, and many other conditions. It is available in wheat or cereals germ, whole grain products, green leafy vegetables, milk, eggs, all whole, raw or sprouted seeds and nuts. Its deficiency can lead to sterility in men and repeated abortions in women, degenerative developments in the coronary system, strokes and heart disease.

The official estimated requirement of this vitamin is 15 international units. Expert nutritionist estimate the actual requirement at 100 to 200 I.U. a day. The therapeutic doses are from 200 to 2400 I.U. daily. It is beneficial in the treatment of various forms of paralysis, diseases of the muscles, arteriosclerosis heart disease by diluting blood vessels. It prevents formation of scars in burns and post-operation healing. It protects against many environmental poisons in air, water and food. It also has a dramatic effect on the reproductive organs and prevents miscarriage, increases male and female fertility and helps to restore male potency.

VITAMIN K

Vitamin K is necessary for the proper clotting of blood, prevention of bleeding and normal liver functions. It aids in reducing excessive menstrual flow. This vitamin is contained in egg yolk, cow's milk, yogurt, alfalfa, green and leafy vegetables, spinach, cauliflower, cabbage and tomato. Its deficiency can lead to sufficient bile salts in the intestines, colitis, lowered vitality and premature ageing.

Chinese Herbs

Chinese Herbs-The Modern Counteractant

A General Synopsis to Chinese Herbs:

The fast advancement in the science and technology has no doubt provided mankind with many conveniences and facilities in the field of medicine, but even now we cannot deny the significance and importance of the herbal cure and treatment. Chinese herbal medicine has great antiquity and history with beneficial and curative roots extending back to Zhou Empire, Late Bronze/Early Iron Age at about 2500 to 3000 years ago.

Due to its shamanistic origins, the current form of etiological concepts is the roots of the ancient herbalism in China now days. In the latter half of the first millennium, there was a troubled socio-economic environment was prevailing in the China and this philosophy and idea of the causes of disease in human society related directly to that disturbed environment of the country at that time. During that dark time of depression and distress, people found the only solution of the sickness in herbal medicine to extirpate those unwanted intruders. That laid the foundation of the traditional Chinese herbal medicine.

The value of herbal medicine is claimed to be one of the most important traditions in China. Scientists working in this field have claims that herbs prescriptions and materials contain active components that can explain many of their actions. Drugs have been developed from those herbs and by them the treatment of many dangerous diseases is possible now. These herbs have a history of more than 2000 years old and since then many useful components have been added in it to make it more effective and valuable. It also decreases the side effects and sometimes replaces them completely.

Early Evidences of Chinese Herbalism:
It is strange to know that the early evidences of the Chinese herbalism were found from the graves of an aristocrat and a physician. These persons belonged to the famous Han Era of 202 BCE to 220 CE.

Valuable medical data and literature of herbalism were found from the grave of the Han aristocrat at a place named Mawagdui in 1973. The medical data was written on silk scrolls. It is very interesting to know that the person was buried in 168 BCE which proves that this valuable medical information and herbal formulas are more than 2000 years old and were used effectively by the people of that time. The herbal literature was based on two hundred and forty seven substances used by the people to cure different diseases.

Very important pharmaceutical data and prescriptions based on herbology was found from the tomb of Han Physician in Wu-Wei county, Kansu province. The grave contained 92 wooden bamboo slips, providing herbal data and medical records included a list of some thirty prescriptions about a hundred drugs.

History of Traditional Chinese Medicine and its Expansion:

Traditional Chinese Medicine (TCM) has a long history. Almost 2000 years ago, canon of medicine was produced in China which is still in existence. This book discussed the experiences, treatments and theories of medicine in full detail. This book laid the foundation of the theories of TCM. This book with its valuable prescriptions was handed down to the Han Dynasty in 221 B.C. it discusses the 365 kinds of drugs and pharmaceutical knowledge from every aspect.

After that in 300 A.D there was a famous eastern doctor Zhang Zhongjing. He gave a systematic and methodical study to the Canon of Acupuncture and problems in medical. He also gave a thorough study to the other valuable prescriptions of that time too and at last he wrote a book 'Treastise on Ferbile Diseases and Miscellaneous Diseases'. It includes the analysis, diagnosis and treatment of different diseases. Later that book was divided in to two parts: Ferbile diseases and Synopsis of Prescriptions of Golden Chamber. Both have 113 and 262 prescriptions respectively. It also laid the foundation of the clinical medicine and is considered to be a great achievement in this field. It is also known as the earliest ancestor of all other books in the study of herbal prescriptions.

Furthermore the contribution of Huang Fumi (215-282 A.D) is also remarkable in TCM. He also compiled a book by rearranging the basic concepts of Plain Questions, Canon of Acupuncture and An Outline of Points for Acupuncture and Moxibustion. This book was regarded as one of the most required reading book in Japan for the B.M candidates. It has put forth a great influence upon the medicine of acupuncture and moxibustion all over the world. Later Chao Yaunfang and Sun Simiao gave an excellent break through to the chinese herbalism by originating new ideas and writing remarkable pieces of writing. The later wrote two books: Prescriptions Worth a Thousand Gold for Emergencies and A Supplement to the Essential Prescriptions Worth a Thousand Gold. Chao worked on Etiology and his notions still exist in the TCM. More attention was paid on TCM in Song Dynasty and the time of a great physician and pharmacologist, Li Shizhen.

Development in Chinese Herbalism:

After that there was a rapid development in the field of herbal medicine in china. It increased to a level of therapeutic sophistication. With the excellent work of Taohong Jing and his workers there was a remarkable advancement in herbalism in China.

By 1596, the Ben Cao Gang Mu of the Ming medical literatus Li Shizhen demonstrated the apex of Chinese herbalism. Then in the centuries of Imperial Era, Chinese herbal medicine continued to develop. Despite of many hindrances this field continued to develop in a very successful way and now if people wants to get a more natural approach towards the herbalism they definitely concerned the herbal data of China.

Now days this subject of Chinese medicine has became very popular among the world and in Australia, The University of Technology in Sydney introduced it as a separate subject. It is one of the only few universities in the world which provides an undergraduate degree in Chinese Herbal medicine. It was the second University in Australia to set up a study program in acupuncture.

Treatment of Disease:

Treatment of many diseases is possible through the

Chinese herbal medicines with far less side effects. Following are the few common diseases and the methods of their treatment through TCM. Moreover, the herbal formulas are designed in such a way that its influence on different body parts are balanced by the other herbs and thus each part of body received the desired effect.

Constipation:

Constipation is associated with the uncomfortable movement of bowels. This usually happens when stools pass through the intestine in a slow manner.

Constipation has many causes including serious diseases like depression, hyperthyroidism, and colon cancer. A deficiency of qi, blood, yin, or yang can be a major cause of constipation. When qi is deficient, the person does not have energy which is necessary to move the bowels and the person is exhausted and tired after trying to do so. A good remedy for this type is Shen Qi Da Bu Wan, which has qi tonics like Astragalus (huang qi) and Codonopsis (dang shen). Cannabis seeds (huo ma ren) are a good supplement or addition, since they are a nourishing, lubricating laxative. They are now easily available in health food stores in the shape of hemp seed oil. If there is deficiency of yang, the person feels cold and may suffer low back pain. In this case, the remedy should also contain Cistanches (rou cong rong); the patient is advised to eat walnuts (hu tao ren), which is a lubricating yang tonic.

If deficiency of yin is the main cause, the person experiences small, hard, dry stools, thirst, night sweats, and a red tongue with very little or no coating at all. The medicine for this case is Rehmannia Teapills with the addition of some hemp seed oil. Acute constipation is comparatively easy to deal with one or two acupuncture treatments and herbal laxatives. The most significant acupuncture point for this condition is Stomach 25 ("Heaven's Axis"), located on the navel on either sides.

Herbal laxatives varying in strengths from mild lubricants to strong purgatives can often bring relief within a time period up to one day depending on the severity of the constipation occurs. Chronic constipation is majorly due to a lacking of one of the vital substances, making tonifying herbs the treatment of choice. The herbs and acupuncture points are applied according to which vital substance needs to be stimulated or nourished. Fully correcting the equilibrium of the body and correcting the balance can take a time period from few days to few months, with a weekly acupuncture treatment acting to maintain qi flowing through the intestine.

Diabetes:

In Chinese medicine, diabetes is considered to be a condition which causes disharmony in the body called wasting and thirsting syndrome. Diabetic can often experience severe thirst and hunger along with lose of weight .There are many herbs. One Chinese herb that has shown beneficial effects in the treatment of diabetes

is called mai men dong or ophiopogon which is used in the treatment. Research shows that it can aggravate the generation of cells in islets of langerhens in the pancreas, which are responsible for the production of insulin and therefore regulate the process of blood sugar in the body.

Stimulation of regeneration of these cells can reverse diabetes in adult-onset diabetics.

Another Chinese herb that has shown good results for people with high blood sugar is tian hua fen or trichosanthis. In research studies tian hua fen has shown to be effective in reducing the sugar level. Other commonly used herbs are astragals and Chinese wild yam.

An Asian vegetable which is also being used as an herb, called bittermelon, or momordica charantia seems to be effective in lowering blood sugar levels in diabetics in researches done in China and in Thailand. In Asia, this herb is potentially applied for treating AIDS, HIV, and hepatitis C.

The Chinese herbal formula Ming Mu Di Huang Wan is used in China for the visionary or defects of eye which are caused due to diabetes. Other herbs are also being used to enhance blood circulation and healing process. It is necessary to monitor the sugar level while taking these herbal medicines so hat the doctor can adjust the dose accordingly.

Cancer:

The major cause of death in the world including china is disease named as cancer. Conventional western style treatment is being used in china since 1960's but the side effects of treating cancer with chemotherapy; radiation and surgery are great. This has led the Chinese government to invest funds in capitalizing treating cancer with the herbs. One such thing is the routine use of fu zhen therapy, an immune enhancing the herbal regimen along with chemotherapy and radiation.

Fu zhen therapy has shown some influence in protecting the immune system and to increase the survival rates , when used in conjunction with the modern chemotherapy and radiation techniques.

Herbal antitoxin therapies are also used commonly. These herbs prohibit and stop the tumor growth by variety of mechanisms.

Kelp and pokeroot are among those herbs which are believed to inhibit the tumor growth.

In the United States, it is very rare that a patient is solely treated with the Chinese herbs although sometimes the results obtained by treating cancer by these herbs are very encouraging and beneficial.

Chinese treatment can be an efficient way of treating cancer patients along with the modern western style treatment.

In china, chemotherapy, radiation and surgery are considered to be the only method of treating if the patient is viable or is in a vulnerable condition because of last stage or seriousness of disease. Conventional treatments with herbs are often done with the patient when there is time available. Although Chinese energetic therapies such as herbal medicine and acupuncture may eventually eradicate or get rid of the pathologic matter, but the problem is that they might take more time then the patient actually has.

Many practitioners in china say that the best result of treating cancer can be obtained only if the treatment is done with both methods. The western style includes the chemotherapy, radiation and surgery along with the conventional herbal treatment, pursuing with the suitable diet, Chinese yoga and therapeutic exercise. Nearly all of the Chinese herbs used today are further divided into three categories: Tonic herbs, toxic clearing herbs and blood activating herbs.

Tonic herbs increase the immunologically active cells and proteins, so they enhance our immune system so that it can resist the disease in a better way. Toxic clearing herbs remove the toxic and germs of waste products from the destruction of germs and tumors. So

these herbs are providing cleaning action. Blood activating herbs reduce the coagulation and inflammatory reactions which are directly associated with the immune system. So they control the reaction of the immune system. Herbal therapy in cancer treatment can increase appetite, reduce nausea and vomiting, and increase stress.

Acne:

Acne is a skin disease usually common among people who are between 25 years to 45 years of age.

Traditional Chinese medicines see acne as a result of environmental heat. The name used for acne in Chinese medicine is "*fei feng fen ci*", or "lesion of the lung wind". Lungs are very important organs in our body and according to the Chinese theory our skin is totally dependent on our lungs to gain beneficial ingredients from our food like water and grain. It helps to keep our skin smooth and fresh. When the lungs and digestive system malfunction, the disorder can occur. In this case any sort of high fat diet can increase this problem. This overall imbalance in the Chinese terms can cause acne.

Traditional Chinese medicine generally classifies acne into three main categories: the blood-heat type, the phlegm-accumulation type and the toxic-heat type.

Blood heat type:

The main symptoms are red papules, tubercles, acnes and inflammatory infiltration around them, and these conditions are usually followed by burning sensation and the tip of tongue gets red. Its therapeutic treatment includes Clearing away pathogenic heat and cooling of blood. the suggested treatment used is Decoction of loquat leaf for clearing the lung path with some additional ingredients.

Phlegm-accumulation:

Main symptoms and signs: Skin lesion is mainly accompanied by acne, in durative acne and cystic acne, along with white and greasy fur on the tongue and slippery pulse. Therapeutic principle includes decreasing phlegm, resolving masses, regulating the ying system and eradicating pathogenic heat.
The Suggested formula used is Two Old Drugs Decoction of peach kernel and safflower with supplementary ingredients

Toxic-heat:

Main symptoms and signs include Malar flush, scattered inflammatory nodules, acne, abscesses and furuncles on the face, associated with red tongue with yellow fur and slippery and rapid pulse.

Therapeutic principle includes removal of pathogenic heat and toxic materials, and cooling the blood and resolving masses.

Suggested treatment includes Antiphlogistic Decoction of Five Drugs with supplementary ingredients.

Depression:

Depression is the most complex sort of disease among all. It has many causes to occur e.g. if a person's self esteem is hurt or the mood is varying etc. it may also be caused due to chronic pain, chronic fatigue, normal grief, vitamin B12 deficiency anemia, foliate deficiency anemia, viral disease, connective tissue/collagen disorders (arthritis), an organic brain disorder, drug side-effects, cancer, and endocrine abnormalities along with endless other causes. Chinese medicine can help in impairing the depression.
One of the methods used in treating depression in traditional Chinese medicine is the 5 element system.
The 5 Elements are Earth, Wood, Metal, Fire and Water. Each element has its own particular strength, weaknesses, color, sound, etc. the most common elements

in depression are Earth, Water, and Wood.
Cortex Albizzia Julbrissin (mimosa tree bark) is a TCM herb which is used to nourish the heart and calm the spirit. It is used for spiritual healing as well. This is used to get rid of emotional constraints which are further a cause of many other diseases. It not only relieves pain but also removes swelling which is caused due to trauma. The flower of the mimosa tree is also used to calm the spirit and also to relieve liver qi which is constrained.

TCM is a medicine which integrates both the body and the soul or mind. So it can be looked as a viable solution for treating depression.

Intestinal Parasites

The different types of herbs are classified according to its characteristics for the treatment of different diseases. Usually a prescription in Traditional Chinese Medicine contains maximum twelve herbs. With the use of Chinese herbs the successful treatment of Blastocystis Hominis Infection is possible. By using the standard Pinyin transliterations, herbs are named after traditional Chinese names.

One of the most common parasitic organisms is Blastocytis hominis. Many people throughout the world are affected by this (single-cell protazoan) infection. It can be treated through the Chinese herbs if the infection is found in the intestine of human body. Generally, it can remain in the intestine for many years but cannot be treated if no symptoms of this infection are found. Loose stools, abdominal cramping or pain, diarrhea, anal itching, flatulence and weight loss are the symptoms of it. Infection rates of any infection are usually higher in rural and developing areas due to unhygienic and dusty environment. Treatments include the antibiotic metronidazole (Flagyl), a combination of sulfamethoxazole and trimethoprim (e.g. Bactrim, Septra) and the antiprotozoal iodoquinol (e.g. Yodoxin). The patient is usually treated for maximum one week with the herbal formulas. Response to medication for blastocystosis differs greatly, and indication may not improve, even with abolition of the parasite or sponge.

Arthritis:

Arthritis is associated with pain in joints and it can
occur in many conditions. Gout, fibromyalgia, pseudogout,
lupus, psoriasis with psoriatic arthritis,
rheumatoid arthritis are some of the more typical and
common conditions that can cause pain in the joints.
The most common form of arthritis, osteoarthritis, can
be treated solely with the Chinese herbs.

Some strong type of arthritis may require drug
treatment which can be combined with the Chinese herbal
treatment to produce beneficial effects. If a person is
suffering from osteoarthritis then gradual loss of the
protective and lubricating cartilage that allows for
smooth movement the bones start to rub together causing
pain and inflammation is obvious in the patient. The
Chinese herbs used here aim at rebuilding and
restructuring the connective tissue and supporting the
cartilage.

The cortisone injections can reduce pain in some cases
but it does not support the cartilage and bones. In
fact in some cases it weakens it by taking away some of
the important minerals from it. In this case Chinese
herbs are very beneficial because they strengthen the
cartilage and bones along with treating the disease.

How to reduce weight:

China is the largest populated country in the world.
But it is an amazing fact to know that you will hardly
find a single fat person there. Chinese medicine for
weight-losing has a long history of over 5000 years.
Losing your weight through Chinese herbs can save you

from any chemical side effect of a normal medicine. That is the main reason that people are rarely fat in china. The routine use of Chinese herbs and its effects makes the people slim, smart and fit. Slimming has never been in the priority in the Traditional Chinese Medicine (TCM) as it has never been a major problem in China like it id in the Western countries. Yin-Yang philosophy and the five elements is an ancient Chinese theory. According to the research of Traditional Chinese Medicine, people gain the wait due to the unhealthy interaction of Yin-Yang and the disturbances in the balance of body organ functions.

Scientists say that when you eat the following process takes place in your body: the food is digested, the nutrients are absorbed and the waste material is extracted from your body. If there is an imbalance in any of these processes it may lead to the gaining of weight due to the retention of water, fat or food. As mentioned above that slimming is not the major focus in the field of Chinese herbal medicine, however there are many people who worked on it and claims to have a weight reducing formula using Chinese herbs.

In fact two Chinese herbal medicines for reducing weight were even banned in China because it was debated that a banned substance N-nitroso-fenfluramine was mixed in those herbal weight loss solutions. This banned substance could have caused heart problems for the people using it. These two drugs were marketed and sold on internet as a natural weight loss supplements but later they were banned in China due to the severe side effect. Most commonly used Chinese herb, Ma Huang or ephedra has also been known to cause heart valve conditions and is banned in the country.

TCM is not in the favor to use any Chinese medicine for the treatment of obesity. Almost all the chinese herbs are mixed with other herbs to treat the fatness. But the combination of different herbs and medicines is based on the metabolic and physical conditions of each individual. The term 'spleen' is very important in this matter. The function of Spleen is to control the transformation and movement of fluids by managing muscles and flesh effectively. It has been proved that the Spleen can be damaged or badly affected by the excessive in take of food. Even if it's the part of your nature to take heavy meals through out the day, you must exercise daily.

Chinese Green Tea:

One of the easiest and safest ways to become slim and smart is to take Chinese herbal green tea daily. Chinese green tea is highly beneficial and processed differently from the other green teas. It helps you losing your weight in a way that it speeds up the body metabolism rate and burns the calories faster. It has a typical flavor and taste. Green tea represses the appetite. The main point to be considered here is that there is no cure in any type of therapy to weight loss. TCM also suggests active life-style and exercise on daily basis to reduce your weight as it is the most effective and harmless way to become slim and smart.

Chinese Herbs and side effects:

It is a common belief of people that around two thousand years back the Chinese herbs were originated in Zhou Dynasty and now these herbs are becoming famous day by day and nee development is being occurred in this field. Chinese herbs are mixed with each other in order to make a drug for treatments of various diseases. These drugs often have side effects and they affect the human body in a very fastidious way. The main intention of using these herbs as a treatment is to affect the whole body and because of that sometimes these effects are negative and harmful for the human body. The reason is that it may have a particular kind of action on the body which is not desired.

The reaction of the herbs directly takes place into the stomach and intestines of human body. Excessive use of Chinese herbs can cause harmful effects to one's body and stomach. Taking herbs before meals can also damage your stomach.

There is no doubt that the Chinese herbs are very useful but due to few herbs can be dangerously harmful for you while using them for remedial purposes. Because over doze of few herbs can be poisonous when taken in and few can lead to allergic reactions. There are more than 3000 various Chinese healing herbs that can be used for curative purposes. However, only 300 to 500 of these herbs are commonly used.

Changing your doze without consulting your doctor might be dangerous for you as various ranges of herbs are used in Chinese herbal medicines. Few prescriptions of herbal solutions include unknown ingredients which might be harmful for your health.

Like other medicines the danger of unwanted reactions and toxic effects remains a main problem for everyone. There is also a possibility that the herbs themselves might not be dangerous or harmful for the human body but there is also a prospective for adulteration and contagion from other toxic materials which are involved while preparing Chinese herbal medicines. According to a published study in Trends in Pharmacological Sciences in March 2002 it was concluded that some Chinese herbal medicines can restrain heavy metals or prescription drugs that could have severe side effects.

Conclusion:

Treatment through Chinese herbal medicines is a well known method used by the people since many centuries. These herbs have been used to treat many diseases and conditions and regarded as the most safe and effective alternatives of medicines. There is no doubt in the fact that these herbs do have some side effects but this reality has not decreased the importance of herbalism around the world.

Chinese herbal medicine is a major feature of traditional Chinese medicine and its focal point is to restore balance of energy, body and spirit to sustain health rather than treating a particular disease or medical condition. The main goal of these herbs is to provide nourishment and benefits to the body.

Longevity Herbs

Articles on Herbs for Longevity

Top Ten Herbs for Longevity

Nov 24, 2009 | By Traci Vandermark
Everyone wants to stay young, and as we age we begin to look harder for something that might delay the aging process. There are numerous herbs that offer anti-aging benefits, but it is important to remember before using herbs that they can interact with other medications. Speak to your physician before adding any herbal product to your daily routine.

Ginkgo Biloba

Ginkgo biloba has been used for years to improve memory and mental functioning, but is now also being used as an herb for longevity of the body and mind. A study in the 2007 issue of "The Journals of Gerontology Series A: Biological Sciences and Medical Sciences," concludes that ginkgo biloba not only helps maintain cognitive function, but it also helps prevent the deterioration of physical muscle and strength.

Hawthorne

You cannot expect to experience longevity without a healthy heart. The University of Maryland Medical Center reports that when given to patients with heart failure, hawthorne was found to be as effective as a leading prescription heart medication.

Gotu Kola

According to UMMC, gotu kola is referred to as "the fountain of life" because Chinese legend tells that an herbalist who used it lived to be over 200 years old. A report from the University of Virgina Health System also reports that gotu kola is used to ward off senility and encourage longevity.

Holy Basil

Holy basil is an herb from India that has a positive effect on almost every system of the body, which contributes to health and longevity. A report in the April 2005 issue of the "Indian Journal of Physiology and Pharmacology" states that eugenol, the active component of holy basil, has a beneficial effect upon the immune system, nervous system, reproductive system, digestive system, cardiovascular system and urinary tract.

Garlic

The March 2001 issue of the "Journal of Nutrition" reports that aged garlic is beneficial to the delay of aging, as well as reducing the risk of heart disease, stroke and brain damage that occurs with Alzheimer's and cancer.

Ginseng

Ginseng is a powerful antioxidant herb, effective in treating diabetes, as well as boosting the function of the immune system and preventing cancer. According to the American Academy of Anti-Aging Medicine, it also helps control blood pressure, a key role in promoting longevity

.

Astralagus

Astralagus is a powerful antioxidant. The Nutrition Research Center states that is beneficial for wound healing, immune system stimulation, and improved heart function.

Bilberry

Bilberry does not have many scientific studies that verify its uses, but the University of Maryland Medical Center reports that it has been used for centuries as a treatment to improve circulation and the strength of arteries and blood vessels, and to moderate the levels of LDL cholesterol.

Milk Thistle

Milk thistle is known for its ability to help maintain liver health. The American Cancer Society reports that milk thistle has been found in some studies to be effective in treating liver disease, especially diseases caused by toxins and certain cancers. They also note that while it is considered safe, you should speak to your doctor before using it.

Echinacea

The 2005 issue of "Biogeronterology" explains that we need elevated levels of immune cells for longevity, and its researchers report that regular intake of echinacea helps the body maintain an elevated level of these cells. These cells also help prevent the development of spontaneous tumors, which tends to occur with the aging process.

Herbs for Longevity-by Michael Downey, BSc

We're all aging all the time. As we grow older, our metabolism–the body's chemical and physical changes from producing energy from food and oxygen in cells– becomes less efficient. This increases our vulnerability to degenerative diseases such as diabetes, heart disease, stroke and cancer. Worse, byproducts of metabolism called free radicals damage cells through oxidation, much like the rusting of a car. The good news is, what studies have suggested for some time is now official: Herbs–rich sources of free radical-quenching antioxidants–help slow the aging process and promote longevity, say experts at the (US) National Institute on Aging in Baltimore.

Antioxidants Battle Free Radicals

Free radicals are thought to be responsible for everything from wrinkled skin to forgetfulness. "Aging occurs when cells get out of balance," says Pamela Starke-Reed, PhD, director of the institute's office of nutrition. "Our bodies produce antioxidants against free radicals, but as we get older, more leakage of free radicals from the cells occurs, creating imbalances." But free radicals can be kept in check. James A. Duke, PhD, an internationally respected botanical researcher at the United States Department of Agriculture, just completed a study of the antioxidants in culinary herbs. "Plants from the mint family–oregano, rosemary, self-heal, thyme, sage, peppermint and spearmint–were the richest sources," he reports. He also recommends a variety of herbs to ensure a wide spectrum of protection. Plants naturally protect themselves from damage by making antioxidants in the leaves to mop up or "quench" free radicals. When we eat these plants, we benefit from the same antioxidants–likely why people who eat diets high in leafy vegetables, salads, herbs and teas are less prone to cancer, heart disease, cataracts and autoimmune diseases common in later life.

Antioxidants for Alzheimer's

One of the most dreaded aspects of growing old, Alzheimer's disease slowly robs its victims of their judgment and memories. To stay mentally sharp, Duke makes a drink he calls "Alzheimeretto." He steeps several sprigs of rosemary in boiled water and drinks the brew or adds it to the bath (many of its antioxidant compounds can be absorbed directly through the skin). Duke says rosemary has about two dozen different antioxidant chemicals that have a similar effect to those in the latest drugs being used to treat Alzheimer's. Other antioxidant-rich herbs he includes are oregano, self-heal, horse balm, mountain mint, spearmint, caraway, dill and fennel.

These herbs also contain chemicals that prevent the breakdown of acetylcholine and choline, brain chemicals in short supply in the brains of Alzheimer's patients. The pharmaceutical agents prescribed for people with Alzheimer's disease are designed to stop or slow the breakdown of these chemicals in the brain and are a hot research topic in neuropharmacology. Duke thinks his drink may contain a greater variety of active agents and be safer, but cautions that he's not recommending anyone follow his prescription until research validates his assumptions. Michael Murray, ND, professor of natural medicine at Bastyr University in Seattle, recommends ginkgo biloba to all his patients over 40. Ginkgo improves central and peripheral nervous system functioning, mental acuity and balance, impotence, macular (eye) degeneration and general circulation. "People who take this herb feel more alert, happier and have an improved sense of well-being. At least 300 [European] scientific studies back up the benefits of ginkgo," says Murray.

Antioxidants Go Wild

As we age, says Weed, our systems slow down and work less effectively. She boosts her vitality by brewing up a variety of herbal infusions. She selects a different dried herb depending on how she feels and what stresses she's under: oat straw for nerves and hormones, red clover blossom for the immune system and stinging nettle and comfrey for the adrenals and blood vessels. These gentle infusions encourage wellness without harmful side-effects.

Antioxidants for All Seasons

Amanda McQuade Crawford, dean of the National College of Phytotherapy in Albuquerque, says, "I'm not so much concerned with aging as I am with optimal health at every age." In winter, Crawford uses burdock root to boost her resiliency and stamina. Burdock is also known to relieve arthritis and provide immune protection—two features that make this herb particularly useful during cold, damp winters when achiness and stiff joints prevail.

You don't need much of it to get these health benefits; just half a root cooked in a stir-fry or soup stock will do the trick. Another herb Crawford relies on through the fall and winter is astragalus. You can buy the dried roots, which are sliced lengthwise and resemble tongue depressors. Astragalus is known as a "toning herb," good for the immune system and prompting the body to work efficiently. Crawford tosses a few slices of astragalus into soup several times a week. She also uses lots of basil, whose oils are immune system boosters and offer antimicrobial protection—defences that can weaken with aging. Crawford uses lots of garlic for its cardiovascular benefits such as reducing "bad" cholesterol.

Antioxidants have become a buzzword, celebrated in everything from cosmetics to supplements. Where does hype leave off and the art of living a more vital, healthy life begin? According to these experts, it begins in our meadows and backyards.

Anti-Aging Herbs for Longevity

By David Cowley

As the Baby Boomer generation is growing older they are getting more and more concerned with staying young. Herbal supplements are becoming very popular with this group of Americans. The Chinese have been researching the benefits of natural cures for the aging process for centuries.

Scientists are applying modern methods to determine the precise effect of these plants have on the anti-aging process. Many of the effects that have been confirmed by modern science have already been studied and popularized in Traditional Chinese Medicine.

Jiaogulan.

Jiaogulan is a Chinese herb also called the Longevity Herb and in Japan it is called Amachazuru and it is used to increase the Superoxide Dismutase (SOD) in the body. Researchers use the SOD levels in studies as a reliable indicator of long life. SOD is one of the body's most important antioxidants. Human studies have showed that SOD levels can returned to youthful levels after taking Jiaogulan for only one month.

Reishi Mushroom

The Reishi mushroom has been used by the Chinese and Japanese and is also known as the "Elixir Of Immortality". It may have the ability to promote long life and improve the healing ability of the human body. It is believed to lower blood pressure, strengthen the immune system, has anti-tumor properties, improves liver functions, improves oxygen utilization, and inhibits histamine release.

Shilajit

Shilajit is found in the Himalayan mountains and has been used by the local residents for centuries. It is not unusual for the people living in that region to live to be over 100 years of age. Shilajit has been used for increasing physical strength, anti-aging, increased sex drive, injury healing, enhances mental function and the immune system.

Foti

Foti also called He Shou Wu in China is legendary in its ability to lengthen life. Modern studies have show that Foti has the ability to lower serum cholesterol, prevent premature gray hair, promote red blood cell growth, and to increase longevity on a cellular level. This herb raises the level of the naturally occurring antioxidant Superoxide Dismutase (SOD) in the body.

The human body can become accustomed to taking herbs over time, and the effects will become less and less beneficial. It is necessary that your body is able to adjust to being without the herb for the effects to be noted when you start taking them again. I recommend that you take herbs for 4 weeks and then abstain for 1 week.

If you just feel that taking vitamins, supplements or herbs to fight the aging process would be beneficial to you then you should always consult with a good health care professional prior to starting any type of home treatment. Always consult your doctor before using this information. This Article is nutritional in nature and is not to be construed as medical advice.

Herbs For Longevity Antiaging Remedies

Tonic herbs for longevity can be taken in small amounts over a long period of time, and are not meant to "alter" or affect any one symptom of disease. The concepts of what a tonic herb is differs in each of the major healing modalities.

The Eastern systems of Chinese and Ayurvedic medicine make use of adaptogens like ginseng to promote a long and healthy life. Herbs that are adaptogens are noted for their effects on slowing the effects of aging by helping decrease the body's reaction to stress.

Western herbalists place more emphasis on antioxidants, nutrition, and detoxification for anti-aging therapy. Herbs such as sassafrass and wormwood are part of the folklore traditions of North American herbalism, and while these herbs are classified as *tonics* and blood purifiers, they are toxic when taken on anything but a very limited basis, making them very different from the other herbs listed here.

Both East and West seem to agree that herbs that support the heart and improve circulation are vital to a long life. Herbs like ginger, ginkgo and hawthorne are some of the most often prescribed herbs and are used worldwide.

Herbs and plants that provide vital nutrition and micronutrients should be made part of a healthy diet just as the fruits, vegetables and grains that sustain our lives. These are the herbs that nourish, protect and strengthen our bodies, mind and spirits. In other words, they are just plain good for you.

Adaptogenic herbs have multiple functions and are also usually considered herbal aphrodisiacs.

Every ancient culture had at least some adaptogenic herbs present in their pharmacopoeia. This is something that is missing and much needed in today's fast paced modern society. Adaptogens are anti-aging herbs that are beneficial to the *whole* body. They never have one specific action, but will actually balance various bodily functions. To put it simply is that adaptogenic herbs help a person *adapt* to the stresses of day to day life.

Herbal adaptogens make up the most powerful elements of the traditional systems that they originate from. Because of their reputation in these folk herbal systems, they have been the most widely studied of all the medicinal herbs, which has resulted in the most mainstream acceptance of their claimed effects. "Why do people still use the other lower quality herbs?", you might be asking. As it turns out, adaptogenic herbs are excellent for strengthening the body overall, but since they're not specific to any one task. Other herbs need to be used to address *specific symptoms* in cases like eliminating parasites, quickly purging toxicity, dealing with acute severe infections and other more advanced states of disease.

What needs to be understood is that the large pharmacopoeia of herbs that is contained in these various traditional systems is great for the herbalist who deals with every form of disease, disability and complaint that people come to them with, but it is much too confusing for the layman (people without herbal training but still have a strong desire for creating positive changes in life expectancy for themselves). That being said, adaptogenic herbs should be used with bit of study into their properties first. I hope this site can perhaps be a place for you to begin this study, or as a source of herb information for you if you're already on the path of understanding the world of medicinal herbs.

The benefits of herbs known to be adaptogens is that they can restore the body to homeostasis better than any medicine because they target and strengthen the *whole* body.

To achieve states of longevity in humans, it is necessary to preserve and strengthen the aspects of youth that tend to diminish with age. A few of these qualities of youth that *tend* to diminish with time, but certainly don't have to are: sexual virility, athletic ability/stamina and physical beauty. Adaptogenic herbs are known, and in most cases proven, to affect one or more of these areas.

In many cases athletes around the world use herbal adaptogens as safe and legal performance enhancers, much in the same was as they would use food and supplements. For example, it was strongly suspected that cordyceps was the "secret weapon" used by the Chinese Olympic team in recent years that has given them such an edge in high level competition. Most adaptogens are also herbal aphrodisiacs. They affect sexual libido either through increasing blood flow to the genital region (while also preventing the diseases found there) or by balancing the hormones of the endocrine system. When hormones are in balance there is also a tendency for the physical appearance to remain vibrant and youthful simply because the body still wishes to be attractive to fulfill its high libido! The best quality herbal adaptogen extracts and whole herbs you can buy online is from either of these two sources

Hyperion Herbs

offers 8+:1 concentrated powder extracts (8+x more potent than the whole herb) which can be mixed directly into smoothies, elixirs, other drinks and/or mixed into food. These Chinese tonic herb extracts dissolve directly into liquids!

Mountain Rose Herbs

Offers bulk whole herbs if you enjoy brewing your own herbal teas. All the herbs on their site are either certified organic or wild-crafted. They have the largest online selection of whole herbs for the best prices. They also offer discounts when you order in bulk.

These fertility herbs will often also do things like reverse gray hairs back to their original colour and even cause bald patches of hair to return with new growth! Many skeptics who don't achieve results with adaptogenic herbs question their effectiveness because they have either not made a *complete change of lifestyle* along with taking the herbal aphrodisiacs. They might also be taking poor quality herbs for too short of a period of time. Herbal adaptogens have long range effects, meaning that they should be taken daily for long periods of time for some of their more valued transformational properties to occur.

The benefits of herbs like these are apparent after months and even years of use. On the other hand, some effects, like the energy boosting qualities of ginseng, can be felt immediately!

Dragon Chinese Herbs from DragonHerbs.com 500 Ginseng Drops -- 2 oz. "500 Ginsengs" is a super-premium full spectrum hydro-ethanolic extract (tincture) of a number of different premium grade varieties of Ginseng. "500 Ginsengs" is a connoisseur-grade product for people who want to experience the power of the finest cultivated and wild Ginseng in the world, expertly blended and extracted as a single product. "500 Ginsengs" is made from a variety of wild, semi-wild and premium-grade cultivated Chinese, Korean, American and Himalayan roots. "500 Ginsengs" is an extremely rich and well-balanced source of ginseng saponins, known as ginsenosides, possessing literally hundreds of these precious saponins, the primary adaptogenic and therapeutic agent of Ginseng, and other closely related saponins (eleutherosides, etc.).

Duanwood Reishi Drops

According to Asian tradition, Reishi is a nourishing tonic, and is a tonic to all three of the Three Treasures (Jing, Qi and Shen), which are the three types of energy that animate a human life. Reishi builds body resistance, and is detoxifying, aphrodisiac, and relaxing. It is widely believed to prolong life and enhance intelligence and wisdom. Reishi has been found to fortify the immune system, protect the cardiovascular system, and to protect the liver. Duanwood Reishi is the best cultivated Reishi in the world. It is grown in a pristine mountain environment at high altitude on natural logs, without the use of any chemicals. It is the most potent Reishi in the world.

Deer Antler Drops

Deer Antler is one of the elite tonics known to mankind. It has been used for thousands of years as a special tonic to promote health and longevity. Deer antler is mainly used as a rejuvenating and strengthening agent. Deer Antler extract tonifies Kidney Yang, Yin Jing, and blood, strengthens the mind and lifts the spirit.

Short term use is believed to quickly build strength and power, while consistent long-term use is believed to re-build and maintain deep life force, preserve youthfulness and to enhance longevity. Dragon Herbs Deer Antler Extract is made exclusively from the "tips" of the deer antler, far and away the most potent part of the deer antler. This extract is super-concentrated. It is the most potent Deer Antler product available on the market anywhere, including Asia.

Chinese Mountain Ant Extract

Mountain Ant from the Chiangbai Mountain high altitude forest has traditionally been known as the "Herb of Kings" because it was used by the Emperors of China to increase their potency and fertility. It is a special variety of ant that has profound tonic properties and is very safe for human consumption. It is now extremely popular in the high end Chinese tonic market by connoisseurs of elite tonic herbs. This is a very rare .

8B Intro Video

8B-Physical Body Health--Diet

(Video Transcription)

Hello I'd like to welcome you to physical body health extended about Diet which is course number eight B. This course was added to the professional personal longevity training program in June of 2015. I covers the content in a new book that I wrote called "Diets and Lifestyles of the World's Oldest Peoples".

And this is really an important baseline component to add to the training program because it really goes into the research that I did about for long live communities around the world. These communities were picked because of the proportion of centenarians and super centenarians that live in them compared to almost any other community in the world.

The communities include Okinawa Japan, the Hansa of northern Pakistan in the foothills of the Himalayas, the Azerbaijanis which are south of Russia on the Black Sea, and finally the town of Vilcabamba in eastern Ecuador on the eastern slopes of the Andes.

All four of these communities have demonstrated over hundreds of years that they provide a very healthy lifestyle and healthy diet for people, and that by following their guidelines we can really help improve our longevity. And in the material you'll study you'll see that the lifestyles are very much in line with the 10 principles but also there were some private surprises we found in the material which I just assumed you read rather let me tell you here. But if you follow their diets and lifestyle practices you will be successful at improving and optimizing your long-term health. So welcome you to this course and I hope you enjoy it. Thanks very much.

Diets and Lifestyles

We struggle with eating healthily, obesity, and access to good nutrition for everyone. But we have a great opportunity to get on the right side of this battle by beginning to think differently about the way that we eat and the way that we approach food-Marcus Samuelsson

Introduction-Diets and Lifestyles

Since becoming immersed in the subject of Longevity and Physical Immortality for the last seven years, I've spent most of my time focusing on the nonphysical aspects of our health and longevity.

What I've learned about long term health is embodied the "10 Principles of Personal Longevity" which is discussed briefly later in this book.

However, the biggest immediate problem which most people suffer in the United States today is being overweight, obese, too fat--whatever you want to call it.

This condition of being overweight affects the entire population and is only getting worse as the chart below shows:

Overweight and obesity

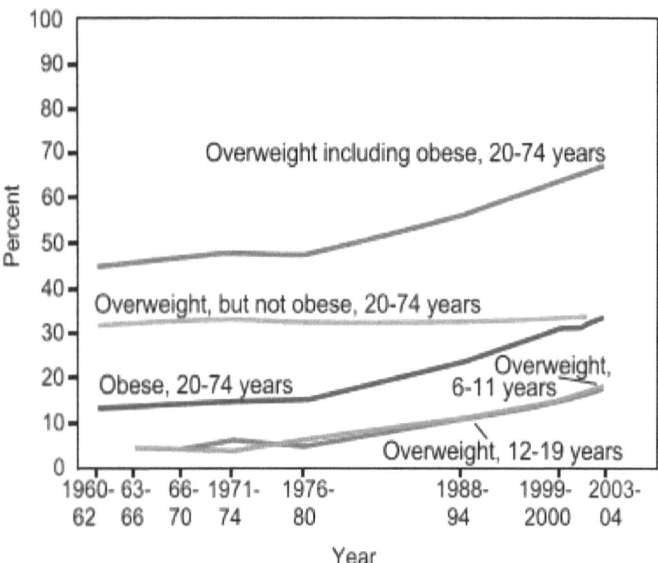

SOURCES: Centers for Disease Control and Prevention, National Center for Health Statistics, Health, United States, 2006. Figure 13. Data from National Health and Nutrition Examination Survey

You probably also know that obesity is one of the prime causes of many chronic diseases including: Diabetes, Heart Disease, High Blood Pressure, and much more.

Most people want to solve their weight problems first before looking at improving their long term health and longevity--and this makes obvious sense.

There are thousands of diet books and diet centers out there--so I wondered for a long time--What unique contribution can I make?

It came to me in an epiphany--That I've developed the correct long term health principles and longevity principles-

-but most people will not learn the 10 Principles of Personal Longevity in a serious way until they can see a path towards ending their weight and obesity problems.

The solution is to take what I know about the world's longest lived cultures and teach people more about what they eat and how they live.

These are real world examples--so why not use them?

Therefore, I've been learning a lot more about these long lived communities and this book is a presentation about those communities lifestyles and what they eat.

I've also included comparison matrixes and summaries of what I learned they all have in common.

Finally, a diet and lifestyle program is recommended for those willing to follow these examples.

I strongly recommend that you don't make any major diet or lifestyle changes according to this book unless you have consulted your Doctor and/or additional certified Diet and Nutrition Professionals.

Hope you enjoy the book and it leads you to our full Longevity training program on the 10 Principles.

The Worlds Longest Lived Communities

I've avoided the subject of the best longevity diets for years since there are thousands of diets out there and I didn't feel I had anything new to present on the subject.

However, I recently spent more time reading about the lifestyles of very long lived persons and decided that the examples they and their communities represent needed to be shown to the world.

There have been many previous researchers and writers on the subject on healthily diets, but I thought my perspective on longevity might be unique since I focus mainly on successful lifestyles….and diet is part of the lifestyle.

The first thing I did in my research was to narrow down choices for the longest lived communities featured in this book

My criteria for picking long lived communities were several:

- An unusually high proportion of the population is over one hundred years

- The community has a well-defined culture

- Sufficient population so that lifestyles and eating habits are a common "Standard" model

- Fairly isolated communities which haven't been too "contaminated" by Western Cultures

The result was a decision to focus on these four communities around the world:

- Okinawa, Japan- This island has a very healthy lifestyle and has been extensively studied for their longevity. Estimate 1.3 million population 2015.

- The Republic of Abkhazia next to southern Russia. Population of 243,000 in 2012 census. A 1970 census had established Abkhazia, then an autonomous region within Soviet Georgia, as the longevity capital of the world. Very many persons over 100 years of age and even into 120-130 age range.

- Vilcabamba, Ecuador-This small community in the mountains of Ecuador is also known as "The Valley of Longevity". Population around 7,000 persons and a very high proportion of persons living to 130-140 years old

- The Hunza People of Pakistan-In far northern Pakistan at an elevation of 8,200 feet have many people over one hundred and persons who are 130-150 years old. An estimated population of 60,000

****

In the next Chapter we will review the Okinawa lifestyle…..

Okinawa Lifestyle

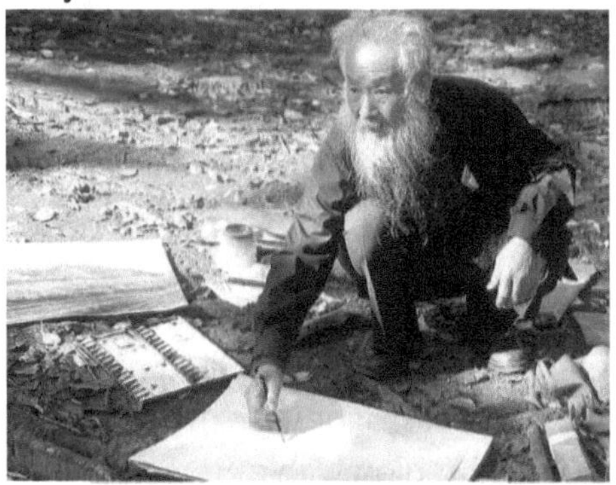

Okinawans have great respect for each other and the elderly:

•	One most prominent custom on Okinawa is bowing. Bowing is an Okinawan greeting...having the same meaning as shaking hands in America. It also shows respect. The deeper the bow, the greater the respect. Normally, one would not bow deeply to a shopkeeper when making a purchase...nor would it be acceptable to merely nod to a person of honor. You will find that Okinawans do not often shake hands. If in doubt, by all means bow.

•	Other Okinawan customs deal with matters of courtesy. First, show respect for the elderly, as they have an exalted place in Okinawan society. Second, you should not walk into Japanese homes, shrines or temples wearing shoes. If you see a tatami (grass) mat, it is usually a clue to take your shoes off. When in doubt, observe our hosts and do as they do. Generally, you do not have to leave a tip at restaurants, hotels, bars or in taxicabs.

Extract of an article from theguardian.com (Wilson, 2001)

So what are the Okinawans doing right? The simple answer is, of course, that they are living a depressingly healthy lifestyle. They don't get drunk every night. They don't eat loads of fast-food and they don't get really, really stressed out over work. They do not chain smoke or work closely with asbestos. Nor do they indulge in class A drugs, a couch-potato lifestyle and the belief that swallowing their anger/grief/fear/panic, packing it all down and screwing the lid on tight is a good way to deal with the bad times. Oh, and they don't live all alone in their old age in 25-storey blocks of flats with a half-dead cat and no visitors from one day to the next.

No - as you may have guessed, the Okinawans (at least the older ones, who've not yet been tainted by western society) are regular paragons of clean, healthy, spiritually-sound living. They eat well, they eat little, they're surrounded by lots of loving family members and they're well into their martial arts and meditation.

What makes their prescription for longevity interesting, however, is in the detail. For a start, the soya. These people eat a lot of soya, and it clearly does them no harm whatsoever, even if it's not keeping them alive. Then there's all the carbohydrate - they get about two thirds of their calories from it. So forget about Hollywood's high-protein, low-carb "zone" diet and those half-baked theories that we're hunter gatherers and poorly suited to eating the fruits of agriculture: you finish your sandwich, love. Some other tips from Okinawa: eat up your sweet potatoes and your watermelon (surely a completely useless fruit?). The Okinawans, who speak a language similar to ancient Japanese, can't get enough of them.

****

We will discuss Okinawan's diet more in the next chapter

Okinawa Diet

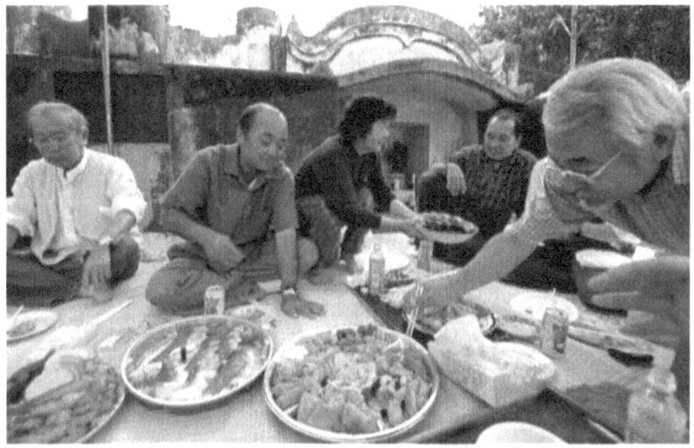

People from the Ryukyu Islands (of which Okinawa is the largest) have a life expectancy among the highest in the world, although the male life expectancy rank among Japanese prefectures has plummeted in recent years.

The traditional diet of the islanders contains 30% green and yellow vegetables. Although the traditional Japanese diet usually includes large quantities of rice, the traditional Okinawa diet consists of smaller quantities of rice; instead the staple is the purple-fleshed Okinawan sweet potato. The Okinawan diet has only 30% of the sugar and 15% of the grains of the average Japanese dietary intake.

The traditional diet also includes a tiny amount of fish (less than half a serving per day) and more in the way of soy and other legumes (6% of total caloric intake). Pork is highly valued, and every part of the pig is eaten, including internal organs. However, pork is primarily only eaten at monthly festivals and the daily diet is almost entirely plant based

Between a sample from Okinawa where life expectancies at birth and 65 were the longest in Japan, and a sample from Akita Prefecture where the life expectancies were much shorter, intakes of calcium, Iron and vitamins A, B1, B2, C, and the proportion of energy from proteins and fats were significantly higher in Okinawa than in Akita. And intakes of carbohydrates and salt were lower in Okinawa than in Akita.

The quantity of pork consumption per person a year in Okinawa is larger than that of the Japanese national average. For example, the quantity of pork consumption per person a year in Okinawa in 1979 was 7.9 kg (17 lb) which exceeded by about 50% that of the Japanese national average.

The dietary intake of Okinawans compared to other Japanese circa 1950 shows that Okinawans consumed:

- fewer total calories (1785 vs 2068)

- less polyunsaturated fat (4.8% of calories vs. 8%)

- less rice (154 grams vs 328g)

- significantly less wheat, barley and other grains (38 g vs. 153g)

- less sugars (3g vs. 8g)

- more legumes (71g vs 55g)

- significantly less fish (15g vs 62g)

- significantly less meat and poultry (3g vs 11g)

- less eggs (1g vs 7 g)

- less dairy (<1g vs 8 g)

- much more sweet potatoes (849g vs 66g)

- less other potatoes (2g vs 47)

- less fruit (<1g vs 44g)

- no pickled vegetables (0g vs 42)

In short, the Okinawans circa 1950 ate sweet potatoes for 849 grams of the 1262 grams of food that they consumed, which constituted 69% of their total calories.

An Okinawan reaching 100 years of age has typically had a diet consistently averaging about one calorie per gram of food and has a BMI of 20.4 in early adulthood and middle age·

****

Next we move to Abkhazia next to Southern Russia to learn about who they are and their lifestyle

Abkhazia Lifestyle

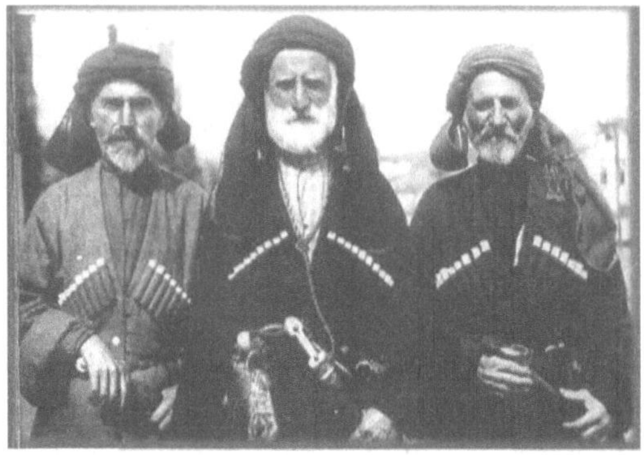

Most of the information about the lifestyle of Abkasian people is taken from the article Abkhazia: Ancients of the Caucasus, by John Robbins (Robbins)

 "Certainly no area in the world," Leaf wrote, "has the reputation for long-lived people to match that of the Caucasus in southern Russia." And in all the Caucasus, the area most renowned for its extraordinary number of healthy centenarians (people above the age of 100) was Abkhazia (pronounced "ab-KAY-zha"). A 1970 census had established Abkhazia, then an autonomous region within Soviet Georgia, as the longevity capital of the world. "We were eager to see the centenarians," Leaf said, "and Abkhazia seemed to be the place to do so."

Abkhazia covers three thousand square miles between the eastern shores of the Black Sea and the crestline of the main Caucasus range. It is bordered on the north by Russia, and on the south by Georgia.

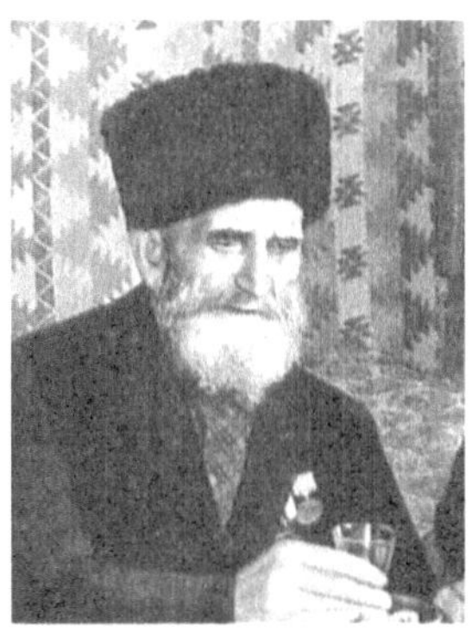

Shirali Mislimov at 168 years old

Prior to Dr. Leaf's visit, claims had been widely circulated for life spans reaching 150 years among the Abkhazians. Just a few years earlier, Life magazine had run an article with photos of Shirali Muslimov, said to be 161 years old. In one of the photos, Muslimov was shown with his third wife. He told the reporter that he had married her when he was 110, that his parents had both lived to be over 100, and that his brother had died at the age of 134.

Muslimov had passed away by the time of Leaf's studies. But a woman named Khfaf Lasuria had also been featured in the Life article. Leaf wanted to meet her, and he found her in the Abkhasian village of Kutol, where she sang in a choir made up entirely, he was told, of Abkhazian centenarians.

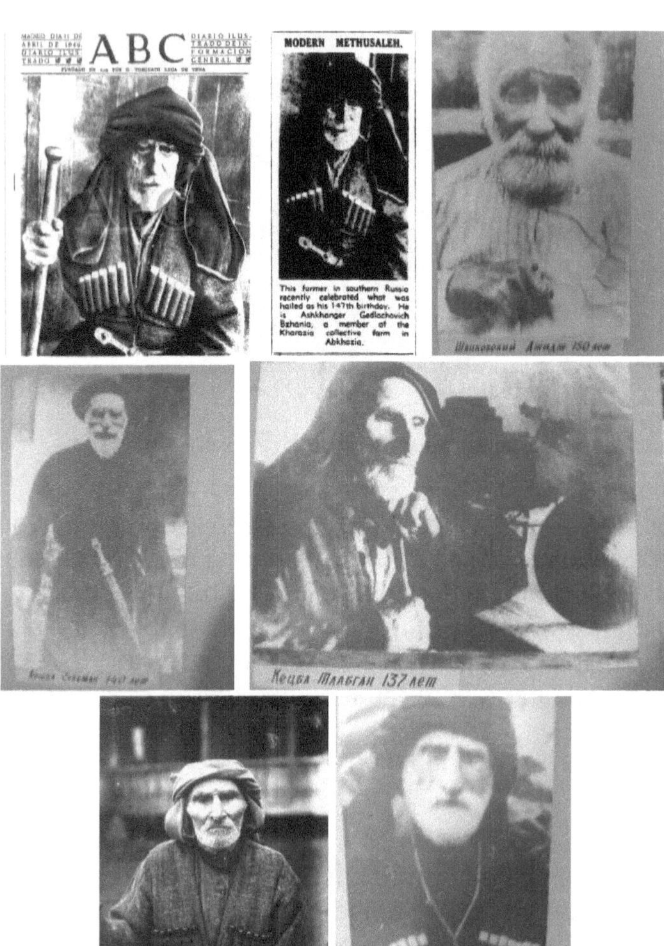

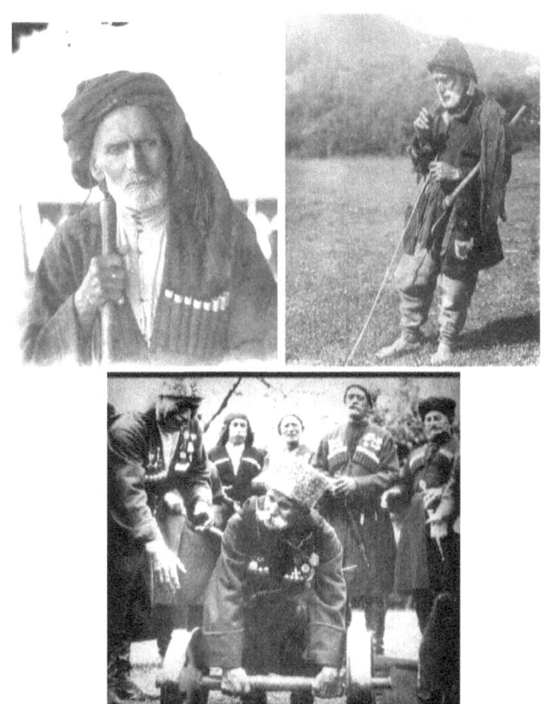

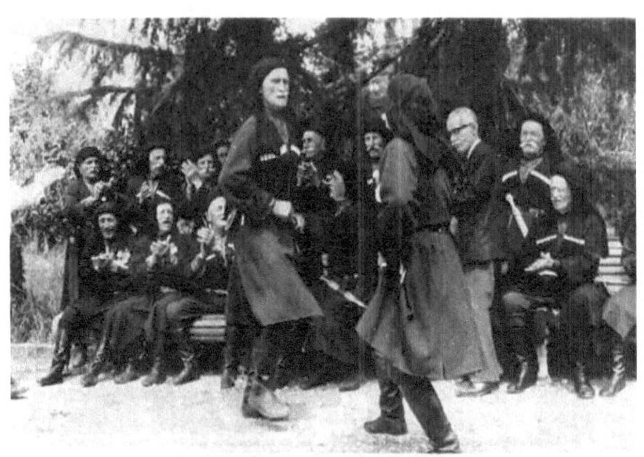

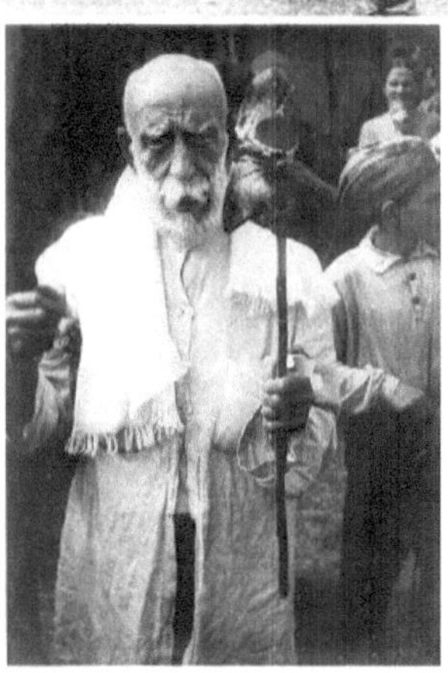

I had a long talk with this diminutive - she stands not five feet tall - sprightly woman who claimed to be 141 years old. . . . Although she carried a handsomely carved wooden walking stick, her nimbleness belied need of it. Her memory seemed excellent. . . . She spoke lucidly and easily about events recent and past. At the age of 75 to 80 as a midwife she assisted more than 100 babies into the world. . . . She described the life of women: "Women had a very difficult time before the Revolution; we were practically slaves." And she ended our talk with a toast, "I want to drink to women all over the world . . . for them not to work too hard and to be happy with their families."

Though he was greatly impressed by this elderly lady's charm and spirit, Leaf did not simply take her word for her age. To the contrary, he went to significant efforts to assess it objectively. Such a task is harder than it might sound, for there are no signs in the human body, like the annual rings of a tree, that tell us a person's age.

After laborious investigations, Leaf concluded that Mrs. Lasuria was close to 130 years old. He wasn't certain about that, saying only that he had arrived at a degree of confidence and this was his best estimate. But he was sure of one thing. She was one of the oldest persons he had ever met.

Everywhere he went in Abkhazia, Leaf met elders in remarkable health. The area seemed to warrant its reputation as the mecca of super longevity. Like others who have studied the elders of Abkhazia, Leaf had colorful stories to tell. He wrote of one elder, nearly 100, whose hearing was still good and whose vision was still superb.

"Have you ever been sick?" Leaf asked.

The elder thought for some time, then replied, "Yes, I recall once having a fever, a long time ago."

"Do you ever see a doctor?"

The old man was surprised by the question, and replied, "Why should I?"

Leaf examined him and found his blood pressure to be normal at 118/60 and his pulse to be regular at 70 beats per minute.

"What was the happiest period of your life?" Leaf asked.

"I feel joy all my life. But I was happiest when my daughter was born. And saddest when my son died at the age of one year from dysentery."

Among the others Leaf met were a delightful trio of gentlemen who, like many elderly Abkhazians, were still working despite their advanced age. They were Markhti Tarkhil, whom Leaf believed to be 104; Temur Tarba, who was apparently 100; and Tikhed Gunba, a mere youngster at 98. All were born locally. Temur said his father died at 110, his mother at 104, and an older brother just that year at 109. After a short exam, Leaf said that Temur's blood pressure was a youthful 120/84, and his pulse was regular at a rate of 69.

The old fellows clowned around constantly, joking and teasing each other and Leaf. While he was checking pulses and blood pressures the other two would shake their heads in mock sadness at the one being examined, saying "Bad, very bad!" They never seemed to tire of friendly joking, always finding new ways to have fun. Leaf was impressed by their sharp minds, high spirits, and relentless sense of humor.

Like many of the elders in Abkhazia, regardless of the weather, these men swam daily in cold mountain streams. One day, Leaf accompanied Markhti Tarkhil on his morning plunge and was astonished by the vitality and physical agility of the 104-year-old. It was a steep and rugged half-mile climb down from the road to the river, but Markhti moved with confident speed and agility. Seeing Markhti take off down the slope, Leaf, a physician coming from a society where elders have thin and fragile bones, was concerned that the older man might fall, and thought he should accompany Markhti down the hill and see to it that he didn't slip. But he was unable to do so, because he couldn't keep up with the pace of the far older man, who as it turned out never lost his footing. Later, Leaf learned from the regional doctor that there is no osteoporosis among the active elders, and that fractures are rare.

When Markhti arrived at the riverbank, he stripped and waded out into the stream, immersing his entire body in the cold water. A young guide Leaf had brought with him from Moscow also stripped and began wading into the water, but immediately jumped out, exclaiming that the water was far too cold.

After bathing in the cold water for some time, Markhti got out, dried himself off, put on his clothes, and proceeded to climb swiftly back up the rugged slope, with Leaf, who was a half-century younger and who considered himself physically fit, once again struggling to keep up.

Are They Really That Old?

After Leaf's articles in National Geographic appeared, however, a heated controversy developed over the validity of the ages claimed by some Abkhazians. When people say they are 140 or 150 years old, this naturally raises eyebrows. When the Soviet press announced that Shirali Muslimov was 168 years old, and the government commemorated the assertion by putting his face on a postage stamp, knowledgeable scientists around the world were skeptical.

How old, in fact, are the oldest Abkhazians? No one knows with absolute certainty. In the days when these elders were born, probably less than one-tenth of 1 percent of the world's population was keeping written birth records. When birth records are lacking or questionable, as they are in almost all cases of people born prior to 1920 in regions like the Caucasus, contemporary researchers have had to be creative in developing methods to appraise the ages of elders. Many volumes have been written about the enterprising techniques that have been employed in the effort, and probably an equal number of scholarly volumes have been written critiquing these techniques. It has been a difficult task.

Probably the foremost skeptic about the extremely old ages sometimes claimed for elders in the Caucasus was a geneticist from Soviet Georgia named Zhores A. Medvedev, an expert in the methodologies used in the effort to arrive at accurate age verifications in Abkhazia and elsewhere in the Caucasus. Medvedev's articles expressing his doubts received a great deal of attention when they were published in the scientific journal The Gerontologist shortly after Leaf's articles appeared in National Geographic. (Gerontology is the study of the changes and associated problems in the mind and body that accompany aging.) In these articles, Medvedev presented convincing evidence that the claims that people were regularly living past the age of 120 were not to be trusted. At the same time, though, he recognized that unusual longevity in the region was a genuine reality, and that the area was indeed home to an inordinate number of extremely healthy elders.

My interest in longevity in Abkhazia, however, doesn't depend on whether any specific individuals have reached ages beyond 120. Perhaps none have, but I don't find the question to be particularly important. What makes these people fascinating to me is the fact that an extraordinary percentage of Abkhazians have lived to ripe old ages while retaining their full health and vigor. What I find remarkable is the high degree of physical and mental fitness commonly found among the elders in Abkhazia, and their obvious joy in life.

****

What do these really old people in Abkhazia eat? Let's find out...

Abkhazia Diet

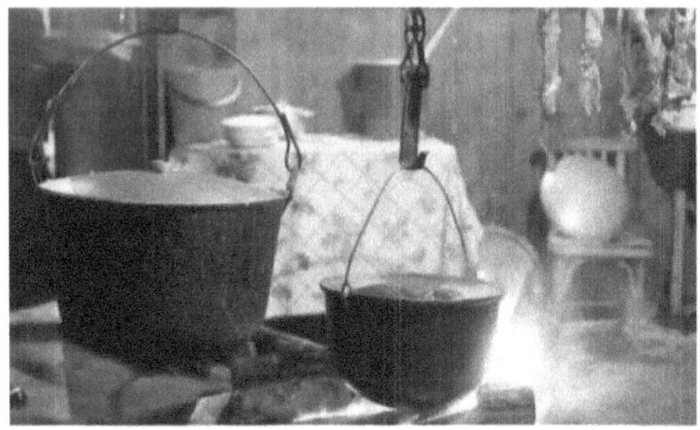

Much of the information on the Abkhazia Diet is taken from the article "Nutrition for Longevity by Dr. Farid Alakbarli (Alakbarli)

The typical diet of Azerbaijani villagers consists primarily of eggs, cheese, butter, yogurt, milk, curds (shor), sour cream, bread, various vegetables, fruits and herbs. They are used to eating soup made of yogurt and greens (dovgha) along with various soups made with beans, peas and grains. In the olden days, people who enjoyed longevity did not eat very much bread or products made of flour.

Animal Fat Consumption
Historically, Azerbaijanis eat fairly large amounts of animal fat, which is considered by modern scientists to be the "No. 1 Killer." Why then has this slayer not visited upon the centenarians from villages of the Lerik district in

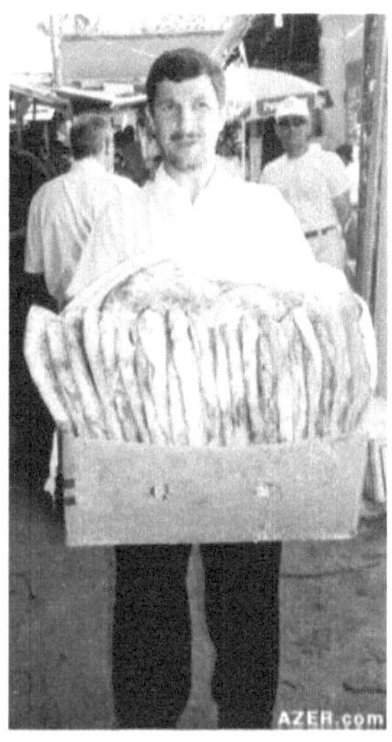

Azerbaijan, where quite a number of residents live beyond 120 years old?

Animal fat is fairly harmless to Azerbaijanis because they follow nutritional guidelines set forth by the physicians of medieval Azerbaijan who insisted that there is no such thing as completely healthy or unhealthy foodstuffs. Rather, these properties are determined a great deal by the quantity that is consumed and the way food is combined.

For example, according to the "Book of Medicine" (Tibbnama, 1712) you can consume animal fat, but you shouldn't overdo it, and you must counter the effects of fat by eating fresh vegetables and greens like spinach, celery, dill, onions, spring onions, coriander, mint, basil, tarragon and parsley. Modern scientists confirm that the food fibers contained in green vegetables and herbs decrease the assimilation of fats in the stomach.

According to modern scientific medicine, animal fat, in fact, must be consumed (though in moderation), as it is necessary for creating hormones and promoting the normal functioning of the liver, heart and brain. If we examine the teeth of a human being, we notice that they contain features typical to both carnivorous and herbivorous beings.

Above: Traditional Tandir bread is wide and flat and made by hand. At Taza Bazaar in downtown Baku.

This fact proves that our early ancestors ate meat, and that the human organism is historically adapted to the consumption of animal fat. However, along with meat, early humans ate large amounts of vegetables and fruits. Medieval Azerbaijani physicians proposed the same approach: Don't eat just meat. Don't eat just vegetables. Eat both and combine them correctly! As opposed to one-sided theories of the modern day, such as vegetarianism, the medieval approach is based on their observation of the biological nature of the human being.

A high level of animal fat consumption is not just limited to longevity in Azerbaijan. Fifteen years ago, correspondents from the Russian magazine "Vokrug Sveta" (Around the World) interviewed elderly people in Abkhazia and questioned them about their diet. It turned out that most of the centenarians enjoyed fatty meat, preferably lamb. As distinct from Azerbaijanis, Georgians drank wine even at the age of 100. However, most people who enjoy longevity in the Caucasus don't eat very much meat in the first place, and they habitually consume large amounts of yogurt as well as vegetables and fruits to neutralize the negative effects of animal fat.

In addition to yogurt and garlic, it is also possible to counter the negative effect of fats with liberal amounts of raw onion, lemon juice, pomegranate juice and with the traditional burgundy- colored, sour spice known as sumag. These all work to promote digestion and break up the fat.

Honey or Sugar?
Even though Azerbaijani cuisine is rich in sweets, traditionally, Azerbaijanis didn't overuse them. When preparing national sweets like pakhlava, shakarbura and halva, they preferred honey over sugar. For example, the Azerbaijani scientist Yusif Khoyi in his "Baghdad's Collection" recommends preparing jams and sweets with honey. Modern science has established that honey contains vitamins, ferments and is considerably healthier than sugar. According to Professor M. Sultanov, the regular use of honey and the avoidance of sugar contribute to health and long life.

Professor John Yudkin of London University points out: "Not fat, but sugar leads to coronary heart disease-the sugar that you pour in coffee or tea, or eat with cakes, sweets or chocolate."

Sugar, if used excessively, turns to fat and cholesterol in the organism. Previously, poor people in the rural areas of Azerbaijan considered sugar as a delicacy and used it only on rare occasions. The standard fare for peasants included dairy products and herbs, not sweets. As for rich people, they preferred honey. According to recipes from the "Tibbnama", all kinds of Azerbaijani halva should be prepared on the basis of honey. Therefore, the harmful influence of "the white killer" that we struggle against in modern society was avoided.

Modern man might think: "Why buy expensive honey, when it's possible to substitute sugar that is much cheaper?" Unfortunately, most of the national desserts in modern Azerbaijan are based on sugar now. But in the long run, such economics are injurious to human health. Muhammad Husein-khan (18th century) also points out that the regular consumption of honey diluted with water prolongs human life. Nevertheless, even though honey is better than sugar, it should not be overused.

<u>Yogurt and Longevity</u>
Since antiquity it was believed that regular consumption of yogurt is the secret to longevity, as it promotes digestion and rejuvenates the organism. The "Tibbnama" recommends adding yogurt to cooked dishes. To promote digestion of meat, it was suggested to serve it with yogurt sprinkled with mint. If you eat yogurt on its own, add chopped garlic.

In Azerbaijan, a popular drink (ayran) is made by diluting salted yogurt with water. This drink is known to lower blood pressure and treat diarrhea. The word "yogurt" itself is of Turkic (Azerbaijani and Turkish) origin and derived from the verb "yogurmak" - "to knead." The medical effect of yogurt is explained by the fact that it contains useful micro-organisms such as lactobacteria.

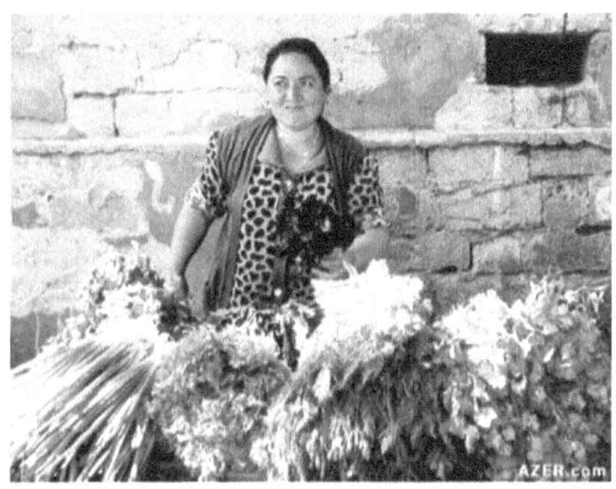

Above: At the bazaar, a woman sells greens such as green onion, dill, cilantro and a purple variety of basil. Vegetables and fresh herbs play an important role in Azerbaijani cuisine.

Since the accumulation of waste substances in the in inflammation of the bowels is harmful to all organs of an organism, normal digestion of food contributes to a healthy and long life. Modern scientists in Japan have also established that regular consumption of yogurt protects the organism from the injurious influence of radioactive rays and prevents the development of cancer.

<u>Garlic - Elixir of Youth</u>
The healing properties of garlic are often mentioned in

books by numerous ancient authors throughout the region-in Azerbaijan, Arabia, Persia, Tibet and China. According to the "Tibbnama", regular consumption of garlic prevents gray hair, strengthens memory and eyesight and is good for the heart. In Tibet, an herbal potion of garlic and spirits was known as an "elixir of youth." In Azerbaijan, physicians used infusions of garlic and saffron in their spirits.

Modern scientists confirm that the regular consumption of garlic lowers the level of cholesterol in the organism and improves the circulation of blood. As a result, all organs are well supplied with blood. For example, a proper supply of blood to the head prevents hair from graying, refreshes the face and improves memory. When blood is able to circulate well in the heart vessels, it prevents myocardial infarction.

Azerbaijanis have combined these two foods - garlic and yogurt - which are typical to diets of people who enjoy the benefits of long life. They chop garlic and add it to yogurt in a dish called "sarimsagli gatig" (yogurt with garlic). The "Tibbnama" also suggests mixing garlic with yogurt. This combination is used as a condiment with dishes made of flour or meat, such as dolma of grape leaves (stuffed grape leaves), khash, khingal and others.

Limit Bread
The excessive use of bread so typical to modern Azerbaijan cuisine can be traced to the influence of Russian cuisine. In the past Azerbaijanis did not overuse bread and flour products. They never had what might be called a cult of bread. Pilaf was never eaten along with

bread because rice was considered to be a substitute for wheat. But these days, many people eat pilaf with bread, and also with national dishes made with dough, such as khingal, gurza, arishta, dushbara, umaj and others.

Physicians of medieval Azerbaijan didn't recommend eating much bread, especially on hot summer days. Modern investigations prove that overuse of bread, desserts and carbohydrates promotes the creation of cholesterol in the organism and leads to coronary disease and obesity. They concluded that overuse of bread is more dangerous than the regular consumption of animal fat.

Note that the national Azerbaijani bread (chorak) does not resemble Russian bread: it is a thin, flat bread, not a round loaf. Another national substitution for bread is lavash, a paper-thin bread - neither of these two types is very heavy to digest when eaten in moderation.

<u>Use of Herbs</u>
Since antiquity, Azerbaijanis have been convinced that saffron and licorice prolong life, refresh the skin and face, and promote health for the liver, heart and kidneys. In addition, persons of longevity traditionally consume large amounts of vegetables and fruits, including apples.

The Azerbaijani physician Yusif Ibn Ismayil Khoyi (1311) wrote: "If eaten regularly, apples rejuvenate the organism, strengthening the heart, stomach, liver, intestine and stimulating the appetite. Regular use of apples prevents heavy breathing and excessive heartbeat in elderly persons. Apples refresh the brain and strengthen its efficiency."

Fruits, vegetables, various wild medicinal plants and products prepared from them - jams, juices, sharbats, wines, dried fruits and spices - all play an important role in Azerbaijan's national cuisine. In particular, hot dishes are combined with various vegetables, fruits, greens and spices.

Modern investigations show that vegetables and fruits contain many micro-elements, vitamins and fibers that neutralize cholesterol. Of course, scientists in the Middle Ages had no knowledge about these substances, but based on close observation, they drew similar conclusions that are being confirmed by modern scientific research.

<u>Tea, Not Coffee</u>
Regular consumption of tea is another main characteristic of people who enjoy long life in Azerbaijan. According to Muhammad Husein-khan (18th century), tea is a healthier beverage than coffee. He points out that: "Tea is a diuretic. It alleviates headaches caused by spasms and cold. In addition, tea cleanses the blood, stomach and brain and refreshes the face. If used moderately, it can treat rapid heartbeat, facilitate regular breathing and is good for the heart. This drink eases melancholy, sorrow and bad spirits."

Modern investigations prove that tea promotes longevity. It contains caffeine, which stimulates the nervous system, and theophylline, which enlarges blood vessels, eliminates spasms and improves the function of the heart. It also contains tannins, which strengthen blood vessels and prevent bleeding. As distinct from coffee, tea not only does not increase the risk of the myocardial infarction but even lowers it, because theophylline enlarges the blood vessels of the heart.

However, one should avoid drinking tea on an empty stomach and should not drink it very hot. Milk neutralizes the negative effects of caffeine. Even though tea mixed with milk is considered to be healthier, it is not popular in Azerbaijan. Tea is historically cultivated in the Lankaran district of Azerbaijan, which curiously enough, is a region known for its longevity.

<u>Cheap, Healthy Food</u>
Although the famous Azerbaijani Oil Baron Haji Zeynalabdin Taghiyev (1823-1924) enjoyed a very long life span, most elderly people in Azerbaijan are not so well off. When analyzing their diet, we see that they eat relatively cheap foods: eggs, yogurt, vegetables, fruits and beans. In addition, most of them don't overeat. Nor are they overweight because they are involved with hard physical labor.

In the past, those who enjoyed long life in our country rarely consumed the expensive dishes of our national cuisine, except on special occasions. Baked goods, kababs, pilaf seasoned with meat and dried fruits were usually reserved for the New Year celebration (Novruz), Muslim religious festivals (such as Gurban Bayram) and wedding celebrations. During the 19th century, even wealthy landowners didn't eat sweets and meat every day because it was considered to be harmful.

Most people in Azerbaijan who enjoy the benefits of longevity actually know nothing about cholesterol, carbohydrates or vegetarianism. They simply maintain the nutritional practices of their fathers and grandfathers, who lived to be more than 100 years old. This reality would seem to prove that Azerbaijan's traditional diet, which has been tried and tested over centuries and millennia, is at least equal to modern theories of healthy nutrition, and may even be superior.

****

Next we move to Ecuador where a special "Vallay of Longevity" exists

Vilcabamba Lifestyle

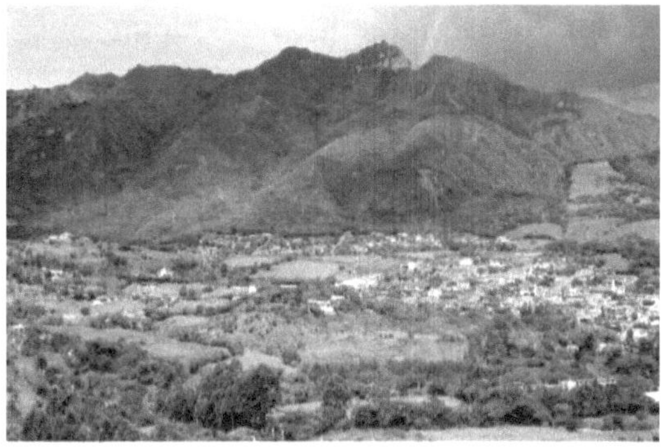

In 1970, scientists researching the link between diet and heart disease visited the small town of Vilcabamba, located high in the Ecuadorian Andes. The scientists included Dr. Alexander Leaf of Harvard Medical School, Dr. Harold Elrick of the University of California at San Diego, and a group from the University of Quito.

The scientists found that the residents of Vilcabamba, who were principally of European descent, had very low cholesterol levels and very few of them ever suffered from heart disease. But more remarkable was the longevity of the Vilcabambans. Many of the town residents claimed to be over 100 years old. A few of them stated their age as being over 140 years old. These ages appeared to be confirmed by birth and baptismal records.

As word of Vilcabamba's "longevos" (very old people) got out, the town became an international sensation. Numerous articles promoted the town as a Shangri-la whose residents -- blessed with extraordinary health and longevity -- lived in closer harmony with nature, untouched by the stresses of modern life. Appropriately, Vilcabamba meant "Sacred Valley" in the Inca language.

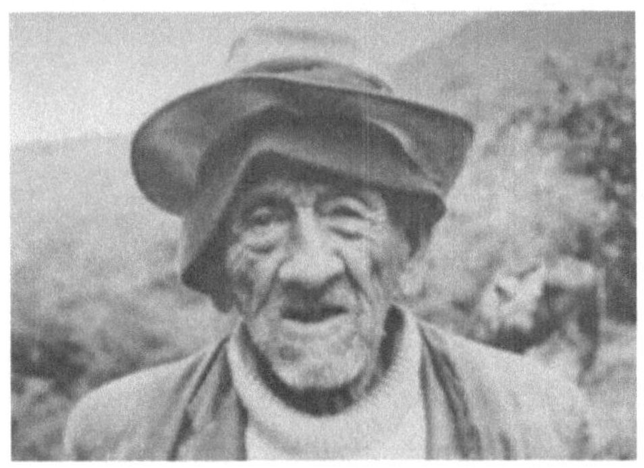

Gabriel Erazo claimed to be 132 years old. He also always wore two hats.

Halsell's picturesque account of life in Vilcabamba emphasized the simple virtues of the villager's way of life. She wrote, "I lived in a dirt-floor mountain hut with Gabriel Erazo, who matter-of-factly says, 'I am 132.'" Halsell described how Erazo stayed healthy by composing poetry in his head while hiking in the mountains. She also wrote of 113-year-old Gabriel Sanchez who "climbed the steep El Chaupi mountain to work all day with his crude hoe or lampa, cultivating a small plot of ground."

Several books published in the mid-1970s further enhanced the town's reputation. In 1975, Dr. David Davies, an English gerontologist, published (Davies, 1975) about his research in Vilcabamba.

There is also the "magical" water they drink:

High up among the surrounding mountain peaks lies an area of primeval tundra, which is made up of great masses of vegetation .... layer upon layer of these grasses and vegetation of many types and colors. In this untouched and uninhabited area, there are also some fourteen lakes, each containing the melt of this uncontaminated glacier ice.

This icy melt is often referred to as "Glacial Milk", a solution of ionically dissolved elements in a suspension of finely ground rock dust from the living parent rock of the mountains through glacial friction. The suspended minerals in this "Glacial Milk" are referred to as metallic colloidal minerals.

Come the rainy season, these lakes of glacial water overflow and flood the tundra, which then acts as a filter for any undesirable heavy metals or minerals. But this humic layer does far more than merely act as a filtering devise. These plants and ancient vegetation had never been exposed to any chemicals, fertilizers or pesticides. The plants are gradually transformed into humus, a rich organic mass that is food for new plant life.

After seeping through these countless layers of humic tundra, this purest of waters flows down into thousands of pools, then into hundreds of cascading waterfalls. And remember this part for a little later, because the countless waterfalls contribute to the extremely high negative ion count in the valley. Finally, the long journey of the pristine Agua Sacrada ends up in the water jugs and homes of the people of Vilcabamba.

They lead active, hard-working lifestyles.

The people of Vilcabamba don't exercise. They don't have to. Almost all of the area's residents are farmers. And the often rugged terrain requires them to hike up the slopes to pick fruits and till the soil on sloping hillsides.

They lead simple lives and have very little stress. The elderly are treated with great respect, and it's considered an honor to have reached old age.

When you lay it all out there, it's a simple formula really. Keep things natural and simple. Put good in, get good out. Work hard. Play hard. And respect your elders. These are the things that have drawn decades of expats to Vilcabamba. But unfortunately many have brought their old habits with them.

Stores now stock many packaged and processed foods. Drug and alcohol abuse are at an all time high among natives, and obesity has found its way onto the town's short list of medical concerns. The locals welcome foreigners and even some of their advancements, but many hope more of them will start to help keep this little-known paradise closer to the way they found it.

In order to properly digest the released nutrients, even with proper chewing, the hydrochloric acid content in the stomach has to be awfully strong. That means maintaining a pH somewhere between 1 and 3. And that, my friends, means having a VERY high acidic level. So how do healthy elders pull this off, while keeping their bodies balanced with a sufficient alkaline content? It's the water!

Laboratory analysis of the Vilcabamba water determined that the unique balance of enriched colloidal minerals in the local drinking water was ideal for promoting optimum human health.

Note the high pH factor:

- ph factor 7.2
- total solids 262 mg
- hydrogen-bicarbonate (HCO2) 136.4
- hardness 140
- calcium 40.8
- magnesium 79.3
- chlorides 10.8
- sulphates 39
- potassium 1.2
- iron 0.03

Now, take a look at the list of the mineral content on the label of the bottled water you are drinking. Does it measure up to what is found in the Vicabamba water? If not, then you are being improperly nourished by the water you are drinking .... If not being outright poisoned!   At least for now and some time to come, Vilcabamba has a good source of clean, sweet water to nourish its inhabitants. This is, unfortunately, not the case in many parts of the world.

****

If you find yourself in Vilcabamba--What should you eat? That's up next...

Vilcabamba Diet

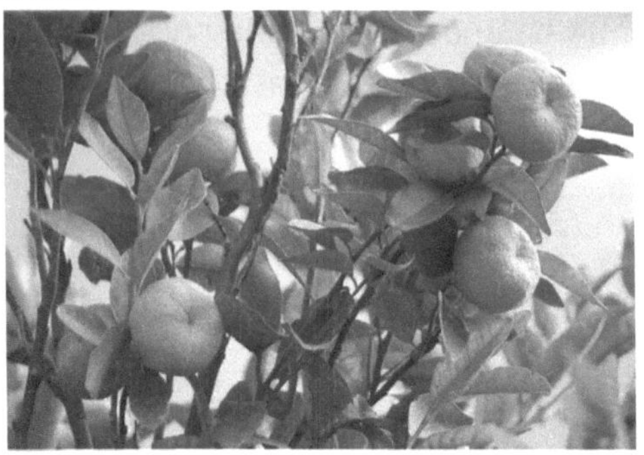

We mentioned the rivers that flow into Vilcabamba, providing water even for the dry season. The year-round availability of pure water allows the town's growing season to span pretty much the entire year. When leaving the tundra, the water also carries with it humus, an organic matter than serves as nutrients for the plants that are grown in the village. As a result, the area's produce has some of the highest antioxidant content in the world.

Keep in mind that Vilcabamba was almost completely unknown to the world until a few decades ago. In fact, until the 1960's, there wasn't even a road that led into the valley. As a result, the area has been protected from "civilization" and a lot of its vices. Chemical additives have never been a part of the area's farming. And, until recently, no packaged or prepared foods could be found on its grocery store shelves.

Residents of Vilcabamba have traditionally enjoyed a diet of fresh produce, whole grains, seeds, and nuts. They eat little fat and almost no animal products.

The book "An Operations Manual for Human Kind" By Paul Patrick Robinson (Robinson, 2011) contains a lot of information about the Vilcabamba diet:

When they prepare a salad they often toss in a few slices of mandarin oranges that grow in such abundance in this valley. The mandarin oranges not only enhance the flavor of the lettuce, but the vitamin C content helps their bodies absorb the iron in the leafy green vegetables. You will also see them mixing some local tomatoes with their broccoli. They have done so down through the ages, this food combining secret passed along from mother to daughter. Now, modern science has proven that these two foods taken together are potent cancer-fighters. Another "secret" ingredient in the Vilcabamban diet is avocado … think guacamole. Once again scientists have shown, after the fact, that the Old People of Vilcabamba were practicing some excellent natural medicine in their plentiful use of avocado in their diet. The natural oil of the avocado works synergistically with the leafy vegetables to maximize the nutrient value of the salad. The medicinal value of culturally traditional foods has always been a part of "folk wisdom" in places where the Centenarians thrive.

Quinoa is called the Queen of Grains. This is cheating a bit. Quinoa, like a number of other exotic grains, isn't really a grain at all … it is technically a fruit. In Botanical terms, quinoa is a pseudo-cereal along with amaranth and teff. It has grown in The Andes Mountains for more than 4,000 years. The Incas called quinoa "the Mother Grain" as eating this food tended to be nurturing and guarantee long life. It is used as a substitute for other grains like rice because of its cooking characteristics.

The quinoa grown in Vilcabamba and surrounding Ecuadorian valleys is a variety called Altiplano, which simply can't be grown in the lower elevations of North America. The quinoa that you are probably used to finding in your local health food store is a brownish, bitterer tasting variety called "Sea Level quinoa." You can find the high altitude quinoa if you look for it, and it's worth the search.

In keeping with the Vilcabambanos use of raw or lightly cooked foods, uncooked seeds are added to soups and stews just as you would with barley or rice. Quinoa seeds absorb water very quickly and become as soft and chewy as cooked rice when added to soups. The seeds also cook very quickly at low temperatures, in only 15 minutes. This is one reason that Ecuadorians call quinoa "little rice."

Quinoa is one of the few foods that has an almost perfect balance of all eight essential amino acids, thus its use as a protein. It was used by the Incan armies in a mixture of quinoa and fat that they called "war balls" to sustain their energy during forced marches at high altitude. So if you want an energy boost and a super-healthy whole grain replacement, enjoy gluten-free South American Quinoa.

Perhaps this is one reason that the centenarians of Vilcabamba have almost always had a diet that was 70-75% uncooked, with an emphasis on salads, vegetables and locally grown fruits. Thus, they remain lean and hardy, not obese and sick.

The Vilcabambanos do cook their lentil beans, and probably so should you unless they are sprouted for salads. One of the types of beans most consumed is the black bean, sometimes called Spanish or Venezuelan beans. This variety of bean is exceptionally nutritious, containing within its dark coating phytonutrients and flavonoids that work together with the natural vitamins to help reduce some of the oxygen-related damage that can occur at higher altitudes. Black beans also contain about 185 milligrams of omega-3 fatty acids per cup, which is about three times most other varieties. It is a nutrient-dense food that goes perfectly with the low caloric intake of the local people.

Their use of natural, organic, unpasteurized yogurt from both goats and cows also provides the beneficial probiotics that might be heated out of the food. It goes without saying that keeping beneficial bacteria levels high in the intestinal tract is one of the best defenses against any pathogens that might be associated with eating "raw" foods.

****

From my research, the Hunza people of Northern Pakistan maybe the healthiest and longest lived community in the world. Let's learn about them next..

Hunza Lifestyle

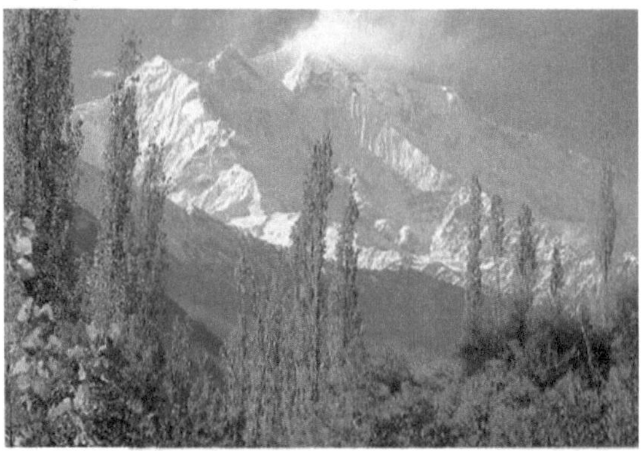

The Hunza people have been the object on numerous studies. The following pages are mostly extracted from the book "Secret to Hunza Superior Health" by Carl Classic 1989 (Classic, 1989)

The famous British physician, Sir Robert McCarrison, visited Hunza at the beginning of this century and brought back amazing reports. In one of his writings, he referred to the nerves of the Hunzakuts as 'solid as cables', while, at the same time calling these wonderful people "sensitive, like a violin string." This extraordinary quality, as well as the other attributes associated with their amazing health he relates to their diet that consisted largely of fruits, grains, vegetables, nuts and green leaves.

Other researchers and visitors to the region have noted similar characteristics and have arrived at the same or similar kinds of conclusions as to the source of these people's amazing health and longevity. But no one has a complete analysis of the elements behind their supreme health and long life. We will discuss these elements in

In 1958, the late Mir is quoted to have told some visitors, "Our people, young and old do not know what fatigue is." As an example of this, it has been noted that an average Hunza man of 80 or ninety years, can walk to Gilgit (a town, 58 miles from Hunza) and, on the same day, return, carrying a heavy load and immediately resume his regular daily routine of extensive hard work. The fact is that each day for every Hunza person consists of much walking and climbing, just to 'get to work' so to speak. Remember, farmlands are sometimes quite difficult to get to.

Producing food in Hunza is not an easy task. This is a mountainous land, nothing is flat, and therefore farming is a tricky and difficult affair. To solve this problem, the social structure of Hunza is one of sparse concentrations of people. The villages are widely separated. And the farms of Hunzaland are built on terraces cut into the hillside and built on masses of gravel which are cone or fan shaped. This design is world famous for its ingenuity and effectiveness. Because, no one area borders any other too closely, no one farm infringes on the farmland of another. Until recently, this structure was sufficient to assure an adequate supply of food for each person. But, in an ever changing world, with an ever increasing population, the ratio of workable farmland to people is becoming too small to comfortably supply the Hunzakuts with food.

THE TEN COMMANDMENTS OF 'SUPERIOR HUNZA HEALTH'

The below 10 commandments align pretty well with the 10 Principles of Personal Longevity. Notice that nonphysical subjects like Love, Usefullness, and low Stress are part of the commandments:

Contrary to popular belief, there is no ONE ingredient that is responsible for the superior health of the people of Hunza. However, there are reasons why these people enjoy the health benefits that they do. The phenomenon is the result of a combination of ingredients, ten elements that work together to make up the "Hunza Health phenomenon"

1 - AIR

Air is the first and most immediate human necessity. Under the right conditions, the human body can subsist for many days without the benefit of food or water, but deprive it of oxygen for only a few minutes and the results will be quite noticeable. The people of Hunza are lucky to live atop a mountain range that is tens of thousands of feet high. They are far away from industry and there are no cars to pump carbon monoxide into the atmosphere. In short, their air is completely unpolluted. It is fresh, clean and totally the opposite of that which we are forced to breathe while living in our overcrowded, highly modernized cities.

2 - PURE AND LIVE WATER

In Hunza, in fact, the only water that is available is that which roars down the sides of snow covered mountains. This is NOT spring water, but as it is relatively unpolluted it is live, fresh and mineral rich. The Hunzakuts, obviously also use this water to feed the vegetables and fruits in their gardens. The special quality of live and freshness of water is contributed to all the things that the Hunza people ingest.

3- WHOLESOME HUMAN NATURAL FOOD

So, what foods do the people of Hunza eat and not eat? Since they lack good pasture land, there are few animals in Hunza, so they do not rely of them for meat or for dairy products. Also, since they are Moslems, pork is not even considered for consumption. Grains play an important role in their diets. The seasons are short in Hunza and they are forced to utilize grains wisely, saving a portion of each year's harvest for next year's planting. For this reason, poultry and, therefore eggs, are scarce, since they do not have enough excess grains to feed the chickens or other birds.

(See more about the Hunza Diet in the Hunza Diet Chapter)

3 "A"- THE LAND

The fact is this: the land we live on and the soil which grows our food is the original source of any life on this planet. The earth (which is another name used for land and soil) is truly the "mother of us all".

Not only are all the ingredients of super healthy communities including Hunza and Vilcabamba organically grown under the most perfect of natural conditions, but the people of these regions improve the soil with natural compost or manure which is produced, obviously, under these same 'ideal' circumstances. Also, the water from the nearby glaciers (which supply the fields) runs over the hills and through the ravines, which are also composed of rich, black soil. As a result, the water carries highly potent, rich mineral sediment to the farmlands which contributes even further to the luxurious and highly nutritional plant growth.

4 - AN ABUNDANCE OF EXERCISE   The kind of Superior Health that has been achieved in Hunza is wrought with continuous, hard, physical labor. But, contrary to what might be first thought, this is precisely the fourth requirement for a natural, healthy and long life.   In Hunza, the whole community, as part of their daily routine is engaged in a great deal of physical activity. Men work alongside their wives; young stand side by side with old. All put in long hours of toil in the orchards, gardens, and fields seemingly without any care or concern for physical tiredness. Incredibly, this work is accomplished

without any aid of modern farming equipment.   And, in addition to work, these people living in such a mountainous area that are forced to hike many miles daily which compounds and adds to the amount of physical energy required of them. This rigorous daily schedule is about the same for the elderly and the very young alike, and includes all the hard physical labors for each group that uncomplicated, primitive life thrives upon. In other words, no one gets any special treatment, but then, no one really NEEDS any special treatment.

5- ADEQUATE SLEEP

A peaceful sleep is one of the important ingredients of "Hunza Health." Sleep time is when your body should be resting in a supremely relaxed state. In this way each cell will be getting revitalized and ready for another day of hard work. Our only recommendation is that you give your body as much sleep time as it requires. You will be surprised to learn that as you change to natural human food and observe the other Hunza Health Commandments (especially exercise) your sleep time will become much more restful and the need for it will decrease. New information points to the conclusion that about six hours of sleep is enough for most people, even those in the most ordinary of health in our modern society. After a reasonable amount of time adhering to the principles of the Health Commandments, you will experience new dimension in sleeping. It will become so restful and deep that you could not have before, imagined it. As for a recommendation on the time to sleep, we refer to the old adage, "early to bed and early to rise, makes a man healthy, wealthy and wise." Seeing the sun rise and set, experiencing the beauty of the day and the natural restfulness of the night will help you to keep in better tune with the ebb and flow of creation's natural time schedule.

6 - MODERATE SUNSHINE   Sunshine is the only source of natural energy for every living thing upon this earth. All life - plant or animal, in the water or on the land, needs the energy of the sun. In a way, an argument could be made that ALL life on earth is merely a FORM of the sun's energy.

7 - FASTING AND RELAXATION   In Hunza there is very little land that is fit for cultivation. Consequently, there is barely enough food for the gradually overpopulating

community. There are times when there is little or no food available to any family. Usually, once a year in late spring and a few days before they begin to harvest the new crops, they will run out of food. During such periods the people go on a compulsory fast. This is the time when their digestive tracts are given a rest and their bodies a chance to cleanse themselves.   As a law of nature, when food is not sustained within the system, the body will start to use its reserve energy by first burning the extra fat cells and then gradually the old and ill cells, converting these to energy. In a society like ours which has become addicted to overeating, a revolutionary but effective method for cleansing the body (especially the digestive system) is fasting. This will also give your body the opportunity to burn away ill, old and fat cells. There are many different methods for fasting. To name but a few, we must include Water Fasting, Wheat Grass Fasting, and Fruit Juice Fasting.

8 - THE SENSE OF LOVE AND USEFULNESS   There have been two important studies in the Caucasus of the Soviet Union (another Super-healthy community called Abkhazia) that relate to how these two senses are maintained in Hunza. The first study, dealing with individuals above the age of eighty, showed that almost all of these people are married and have been for the length of their adult lives. The number of single people who are of advanced age is very small. This indicates that an important element in longevity is the mutual love and caring of a close human relationship.

These two studies are especially striking when viewed in the light of the Hunza population. There the aged enjoy a very high social status, in the community as well as in the family. Elderly people always live with family and close relatives, which often makes for an outstandingly large household. However, even in these large families the elderly are the center of attention, occupying a privileged position. The elderly are esteemed for their wisdom in Hunza, and the young universally believe that this is derived from long life and extensive experience. This makes the aged person's word as acceptable as law.

In Hunza, family members almost always consult the eldest member when making any major decision. This love and respect in family and community, plus the physical and economical work that these people do helps to give the people of Hunza, well into ages over one hundred, a sense of responsibility, love and usefulness. This sense of usefulness is highly important in any individual in order for him to continue to live to these advanced ages. Psychologists have repeatedly reinforced this fact: Once a person concludes in his own mind that his existence no longer has any purpose, at that point he has verified his own Death Certificate. In Hunza, and all their counterpart communities who are famous for superior health and longevity, there is no forced or accepted retirement age. The elderly are NOT thrown out of the family or the community and their sense of responsibility is not taken away from them, as is the case in most modern societies.

9- LIMITED WORRY AND STRESS Anyone would certainly agree that life in a remote, mountain valley, where peace and tranquility abound, would be a little easier to deal with than all the hassles we have in modern life. If we were lucky enough to live in a place where the air is fresh and clean, the water pure and living, the food wholesome and natural, and where we were literally hundreds of miles away from the nearest fear, worry, emotional complication or stress, we would probably want to live to be as old as possible.

If we had the time, we could list hundreds of stresses and emotional pressures that are an integral part of modern life, but are unknown in communities such as Hunza. To name but a few, there is the stress of driving in traffic, the daily stress of jobs, worries about weight (either being too fat, or the new one, being too skinny), worries about paying bills, fear of unemployment, fear of physical safety and security of property, law suits from enemies, worries about health and so on.

10- LACK OF GREED AND ENVY   Greed and Envy are important factors in any modern society which bases the success of individuals according to their relative status in that society. How we measure our status, as compared to our neighbors, is not important. The issue is not whether we are capitalists or socialists, speak one language or another. When it comes to Greed and Envy the result to human health is going to be serious harm.

****

And yes--Of course we want to know what the Hunzas eat...

Hunza Diet

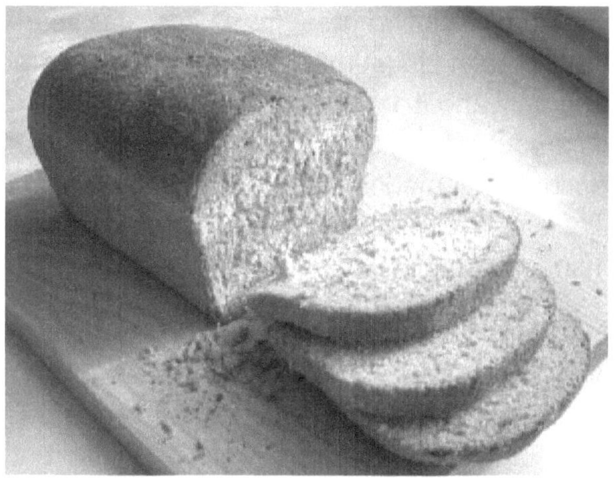

What the Hunzakuts thrive on, mostly, is the famous Hunza Bread. This is made from a coarse, whole grain, barley flour and water and formed into a kind of pancake. Remember, this is WHOLE GRAIN, hand-ground and fresh from a clean highly fertile land.   In addition, they also eat a lot of vegetables, green leaves, fruits, grain and some nuts. Their grain selection includes wheat, barley, buckwheat, corn, millet, alfalfa, and rye. Their vegetables are mostly potatoes, tomatoes, carrots, onions, garlic, peas, beans and pulses. The fruits that are generally available in the region are mulberries, apricots, apples, cucumbers, grapes, peaches, cherries and some melons. It's an excellent variety that appears to supply all essential vitamins in precise quantities.

The diet of these people was studied by Pakistani nutritionist, Dr. S. Maqsood. He found the average caloric intake of the Hunzakuts to be about 1900 (about 2/3 that of an average American). 98 1/2% of this consisted of protein, fat and carbohydrates "from vegetable sources." The food originating in animal flesh or from dairy products comprised only about 1 1/2% of their total food intake. And, this amount is calculated from an average consumption. That means that the animal by-products part of the diet is not consistent, but rather sporadic causing little continual damage.

The most important single observation to be made about food consumption in Hunzaland is that almost everything is eaten raw, uncooked, and just as nature intended. This preference for live food includes every kind of sprout (one of the most 'living' sources of nutrition known).

In summary then, the people of Hunza eat almost nothing in the way of meat, dairy products, eggs, animal fats or processed and chemicalized foods. The only exceptions to this come with what is now being brought into the area from the outside, as "progress" makes its unhealthy advance on the people of this peaceful mountain region.

What we have outlined here appears to be the latest craze in 'healthy diets' in the U.S., but, in fact is the classic "Hunza Health Recipe." Our third Health Commandment then is based upon the knowledge that a community (which exists today) is surviving in a much more healthy way because they have followed (more closely) the diet that the Creator intended for us. The Commandment is this, "Work in harmony with your earth so that it will yield foods for you that consist mainly of live, organically grown grains, seeds, vegetables and nuts. Eat these raw and don't tamper with the way they are given to you."

****

Now let's do comparison matrixes for all of these communities to compare lifestyles and diets side by side….

Lifestyle & Diet Recommendations

Before making specific diet suggestions based on these four long lived communities I decided to make a matrix of both cultural and dietary factors. These factors are rated (High-Medium-Low) Types of foods are also provided in the Diet Table.

<u>Lifestyle Factors</u>

Description	Okinawa	Abkhazia	Vilcabamba	Hunzas
Exercise	*High*	*High*	*Medium*	*Very High*
Naturally Pure Water	*Medium*	*High*	*High*	*High*
Sense of Community	*High*	*High*	*High*	*High*
Happiness	*High*	*High*	*High*	*High*
Spiritual Practices & Inner Peace	*High*	*High*	*High*	*High*
Respect	*High*	*High*	*High*	*High*

for Elderly				

<u>Dietary Factors/Foods</u>

Description	Okinawa	Abkhazia	Vilcabamba	Hunzas
Vegetables	*High-Sweet Potatos, Goya (bitter melon), Shima Rakkyo, Okra, Handama, Carrots, radish, marrow, onions, carrots, cabbage and leafy greens, Soya, squash*	*High-string beans, corn, cabbage, tomatoes, spinach, celery, dill, onions, spring onions, coriander, mint, basil, tarragon and parsley*	*High-Potatos, Mayoko, Payoko*	*High-Tomatoes, onions, garlic, spinach, turnips, carrots, pumpkins, cabbage, and cauliflower*
Legumes	*High*	*High*	*High*	*High-beans, lentils*
Meat/Fat	*Low-Pork*	*Low-Lamb*	*Low*	*Minimal*

Grains	*Rice*	*Buckwheat*	*High-Trigo (Wheat), Rice*	*wheat, barley, buckwheat, corn, millet, alfalfa, and rye*
Fish	*Low*	*Low*	*Low*	*Minimal*
Fruits	*High-Watermelon, Pineapple, Mango, Papaya, Passion Fruit, Shiikwa*	*High-Apples, cherry plums, barberries, blackberries, pomegranates, green grapes, tomatoes*	*High-oranges, blackberries, papayas, bananas, figs, avocados, Citroen, Granadias*	*High-mulberries, apricots, apples, cucumbers, grapes, peaches, cherries and some melons*
Nuts	*Pine nuts*	*Achapa, Walnuts*	*High-macadamia nuts, almonds*	*Almonds, Beachnuts, Walnuts, Flax*

Special Bread		*High-Limit Bread*		*High-Hunza Bread*
Sugars	*Sugarcane (Unrefined)*	*Honey, Sugarbeets*	*Panela- (Unrefined Sugarcane)*	*Honey*
Other Common Foods		*Yogurt, Garlic*	*Quinoa*	*Yogurt*
Common Herbs		*Saffron, Licorice*		
Common Drinks	*High-Tumeric Tea*	*High-Tea, Mountain Waters*	*High-Mountain Waters (Glacial Milk)*	*High-Mountain Waters*
Number of Daily Meals				*Two*

From the above tables comparing lifestyles and diets here are my recommendations for the Longevity Diet which is taken from these real world examples:

1) Drink Pure Water--but not just bottled water but water with appropriate nutrients like the mountain streams provide to the long lived communities.

2) None of these communities are pure vegetarians but they all have very low levels of meat and fish--just because their traditional diets are oriented that way. Meat and Fish comprises only 1-3% of their daily diets

3) Two communities-- the Abkhazians and Hunzas eat natural grain, low fat, and high protein breads with fruit and nuts added. These are Limit Breads for the Abkhazians, and Hunza Breads for the Hunzas.

4) Several of the communities have lots of home grown fruits--of a variety of types. Eat lots of fruit.

5) Sugars are all natural or unrefined sugars whether from honey or from various types of fruits, or sugarcane.

6) They all consume high levels of legumes and vegetables. These types of food are the large majorities of their diets. (Greater than 65%)

7) The number of meals daily are only stated for the Hunzas who regularly eat two large meals daily. My research didn't tell me the number of meals in the other communities.

<u>The Effect of Lifestyle Factors:</u>

In the lifestyle factors table you can see a lot of parallels to the 10 Principles of Personal Longevity.

The principle longevity lifestyle factors I found from my research include:

- Lots of daily exercise--This ties into my previous research that exercise is one of the most critical factors in long term health.
- Naturally Pure Water with mountain nutrients-This was a surprise to me since I've heard others tout the benefits of water but never really gave it much serious consideration
- A strong Sense of Community- The community and happiness factors both illustrate the need for purpose and happiness to make our lives more fulfilling
- Overall Happiness
- Spiritual Practices & Inner Peace--A critical factor I've been teaching for years having earlier found that almost all super centenarians have these attributes which I believe help bring a spiritual blueprint of health down into our bodies
- Respect for Elderly--This relates a lot to the Principle of Life Purpose. People need meaning in their lives to go on living and being respected and asked for advice as an elderly person is important in making their lives worthwhile.

If you have read any of my other books on Longevity you will realize that these lifestyle factors are all part of what we already teach. They show some real world examples which further validate our 10 Principles approach.

****

Next lets look at a new Diet and Lifestyle Plan to apply what we have learned to ourselves…

A Longevity Diet & Lifestyle Plan

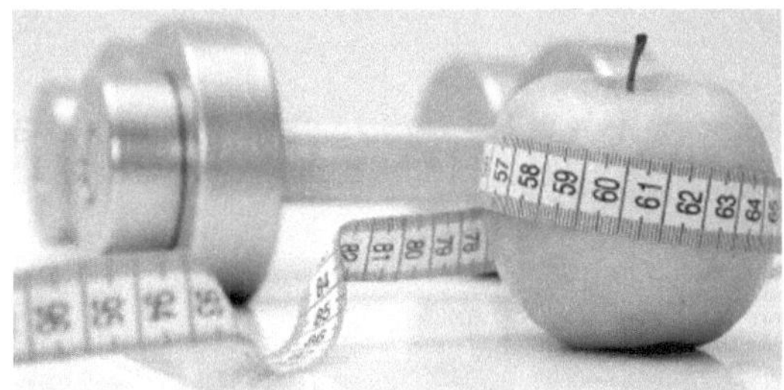

Changing your lifestyle and diet to a new permanent and healthier "standard" or "baseline" is not easy to do.

It is up to your motivation and willingness to follow these steps --and get help from others to hold you accountable.

<u>STEP #1:</u>

Determine what your breakeven level of calories is per day. In other words how many calories can you eat daily without gaining any weight? Also determine how many calories you should eat daily in "weight loss mode".

An example table is below on general calorie levels need by sex and age:

Age and gender	Estimated calories for those who are not physically active	
	Total daily calorie needs*	Daily limit for empty calories
Children 2-3 yrs	1000 cals	135**
Children 4-8 yrs	1200-1400 cals	120
Girls 9-13 yrs	1600 cals	120
Boys 9-13 yrs	1800 cals	160
Girls 14-18 yrs	1800 cals	160
Boys 14-18 yrs	2200 cals	265
Females 19-30 yrs	2000 cals	260
Males 19-30 yrs	2400 cals	330
Females 31-50 yrs	1800 cals	160
Males 31-50 yrs	2200 cals	265
Females 51+ yrs	1600 cals	120
Males 51+ yrs	2000 cals	260

However, the above table may not apply to everyone based on your body type and metabolism.

I encourage you to work with a medical professional to carefully determine your daily caloric needs.

Once you have a good caloric number we can proceed to Step 2:

STEP #2:

Start changing what you drink to conform to longevity community guidelines.

For example--drink healthy pure water--like these old people do from their mountain streams. You may not have access to the streams but you do have access to lots of brands of pure water and you can get recommendations on additional mineral waters.

The Mayo Clinic has determined these average guidelines for the amount of water you should drink each day:

The Institute of Medicine determined that an adequate intake (AI) for men is roughly about 13 cups (3 liters) of total beverages a day. The AI for women is about 9 cups (2.2 liters) of total beverages a day.

<u>Stop drinking all sodas and other diet or sugary drinks. They are all bad for you</u>

Most of us lived dehydrated and we should drink much more water each day than we currently do.

<u>STEP #3:</u>

Start planning meals from the "Dietary Factors/Foods" Table which lists many grains, nuts, and fruits which the long lived communities each. This is in the Chapter titled " Lifestyle & Diet Recommendations"

You should make these types of food the staples of your daily diet.

This includes the various breads like Hunza Bread--whose recipe is given in the recipe chapter below.

The calorie intake you should plan for daily should be less than your breakeven calorie intake. Your daily intake should be the number your worked out with your health professional.

My doctor friend worked out the numbers for me to lose weight. Since I'm a big guy she calculated that my breakeven value was 3600 calories per day. She recommended that I only consume about 2800 calories per day while I was still trying to lose weight.

These numbers will be different for everyone--which is why you should consult a medical and/or diet and nutrition professional.

I also decided to follow the Hunza practice of only eating two meals per day with snacks in between--this is just me-- I'm not recommending that everyone eat two meals per day.

Another factor to consider are meats, poultry, and fish. You don't need to become a vegetarian but it is important to realize that most long lived communities only consume about 1-3% of their diet as meat, poultry, and fish.

Most of this long term healthy diet is going to be grains, nuts, and fruits--so you just need to get used to it.

<u>STEP #4:</u>

Daily Exercise is required. You must exercise every day the rest of your life.

Let me elaborate--In all of my studies of long lived people well over 100 only two factors stood out:

* Daily exercise even into extreme old age

* Inner Peach and/or Spiritual Practices

Each of the communities we cover in this book also have lifestyles which involve heavy daily exercise--and no you don't get to quit when you reach 100 years old.

A basic rule of thumb I've learned is "If you want to live-- keep exercising. If you want to die-Stop".

It doesn't have to be a huge amount of exercise daily. Maybe just a walk for 20 minutes.--but it has to be something.

You can work with a Personal Trainer to develop your own daily program if you don't know what to do yourself.

<u>SO EXERCISE AND KEEP DOING IT FOREVER !</u>

<u>Step #5:</u>

Once you have started to reduce your weight and lead a healthier lifestyle then you are ready for the next and biggest step---

Summary-Diets and Lifestyles

This book is intended as a starting point for improving your health by losing weight and starting to live a healthier lifestyle.

We can best learn from what has worked for others.

The four communities in this book are historical labs which have experiential information on what long lived people actually eat and how they live.

The Diet Steps are just some guidelines to get your started. If you are serious about your optimal health then you should follow the path to take our longevity training too.

The Recipes which are included are designed to show you ways to prepare food as these longevity communities do.

My best wishes to you in improving and taking control of your life.

8C-Intro Video

(Video Transcript)

Hello and welcome to this course on your weight and exercise. I wanted to include this to round out the courses on the physical body as part of the longevity coaching program.

As you're well aware there are thousands of books, videos, and TV programs-everything about your weight, and weight loss, and the importance of exercise. I didn't want to rehash all of those-I just wanted to cover some basic issues as regards longevity and your weight and exercise.

And that's what this course is about-so these things include misunderstandings about how these two factors are related to your longevity. What some studies show about your weight and exercise-some surprising facts as a matter of fact. And then there are a couple of basic concepts. You can talk to people about their own weight and the importance of reducing it for longevity.

And the importance of exercise and what are the minimal amounts of exercise that people can do to help them retain long term health. So my goal is a little different than a lot of people. I'm not trying to get you to exercise enough to go run a marathon. No it's more about what are the optimal levels to help your long term health for both your weight, your BMI, or body mass index, and the exercise you need to do at a minimal level just to stay healthy in the long term Thank You

8C-Physical Body Health-Weight and Exercise

Introduction-Effects of Weight and Exercise on Longevity

Dear Reader, if you are familiar with my work you might already be aware that I promote a lifestyle to help people integrate spirit, mind, and body.

This book is focused on Principle #8—How to keep your physical body healthy and specifically on how Weight and Exercise are related to Longevity.

It is a survey of the latest articles and scientific studies available.

I should also clearly state that I'm an engineer and not a certified medical professional, so anything I write in this book should be taken with a grain of salt.

Terms of Measurement

First let's establish some common terms used by scientists and medical professionals to talk about our weight and exercise:

BMI—Body Mass Index is….

BMI is a person's weight in kilograms (kg) divided by his or her height in meters squared. The National Institutes of Health (NIH) now defines normal weight, overweight, and obesity according to **BMI** rather than the traditional height/weight charts. Overweight is a **BMI** of 27.3 or more for women and 27.8 or more for men.

The table below shows BMI calculations for different weights and heights:

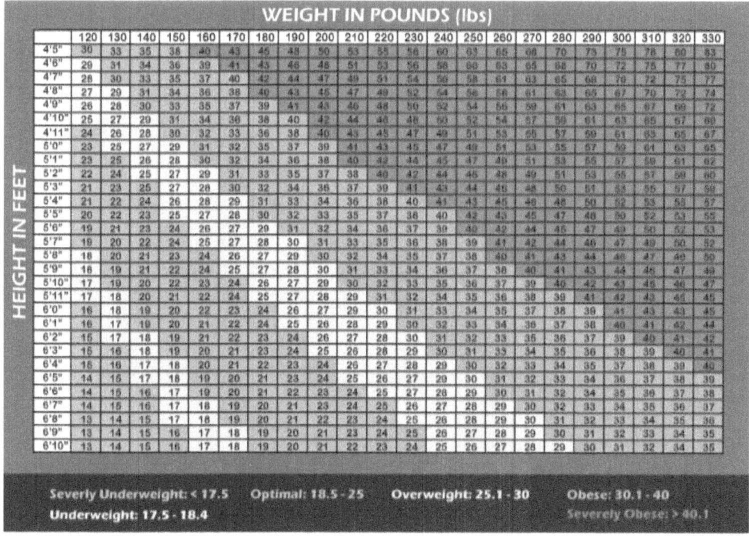

WEIGHT IN POUNDS (lbs)

HEIGHT IN FEET	120	130	140	150	160	170	180	190	200	210	220	230	240	250	260	270	280	290	300	310	320	330
4'5"	30	33	35	38	40	43	45	48	50	53	55	58	60	63	65	68	70	73	75	78	80	83
4'6"	29	31	34	36	39	41	43	46	48	51	53	56	58	60	63	65	68	70	72	75	77	80
4'7"	28	30	33	35	37	40	42	44	47	49	51	54	56	58	61	63	65	68	70	72	75	77
4'8"	27	29	31	34	36	38	40	43	45	47	49	52	54	56	58	61	63	65	67	70	72	74
4'9"	26	28	30	33	35	37	39	41	43	46	48	50	52	54	56	59	61	63	65	67	69	72
4'10"	25	27	29	31	34	36	38	40	42	44	46	48	50	52	54	57	59	61	63	65	67	69
4'11"	24	26	28	30	32	33	36	38	40	43	45	47	49	51	53	55	57	59	61	63	65	67
5'0"	23	25	27	29	31	32	35	37	39	41	43	45	47	49	51	53	55	57	59	61	63	65
5'1"	23	25	26	28	30	32	34	36	38	40	42	44	45	47	49	51	53	55	57	59	61	62
5'2"	22	24	25	27	29	31	33	35	37	38	40	42	44	46	48	49	51	53	55	57	58	60
5'3"	21	23	25	27	28	30	32	34	36	37	39	41	43	44	46	48	50	51	53	55	57	58
5'4"	21	22	24	26	28	29	31	33	34	36	38	40	41	43	45	46	48	50	52	53	55	57
5'5"	20	22	23	25	27	28	30	32	33	35	37	38	40	42	43	45	47	48	50	52	53	55
5'6"	19	21	23	24	26	27	29	31	32	34	36	37	39	40	42	44	45	47	49	50	52	53
5'7"	19	20	22	24	25	27	28	30	31	33	35	36	38	39	41	42	44	46	47	49	50	52
5'8"	18	20	21	23	24	26	27	29	30	32	34	35	37	38	40	41	43	44	46	47	49	50
5'9"	18	19	21	22	24	25	27	28	30	31	33	34	36	37	39	40	42	43	45	46	47	48
5'10"	17	19	20	22	23	24	26	27	29	30	32	33	35	36	37	39	40	42	43	45	46	47
5'11"	17	18	20	21	22	24	25	27	28	29	31	32	34	35	36	38	39	41	42	43	45	45
6'0"	16	18	19	20	22	23	24	26	27	29	30	31	33	34	35	37	38	39	41	43	43	45
6'1"	16	17	19	20	21	22	24	25	26	28	29	30	32	33	34	36	37	38	40	41	42	44
6'2"	15	17	18	19	21	22	23	24	26	27	28	30	31	32	33	35	36	37	39	40	41	42
6'3"	15	16	18	19	20	21	23	24	25	26	28	29	30	31	33	34	35	36	38	39	40	41
6'4"	15	16	17	18	20	21	22	23	24	26	27	28	29	30	32	33	34	35	37	38	39	40
6'5"	14	15	17	18	19	20	21	23	24	25	26	27	29	30	31	32	33	34	36	37	38	39
6'6"	14	15	16	17	19	20	21	22	23	24	25	27	28	29	30	31	32	34	35	36	37	38
6'7"	14	15	16	17	18	19	20	21	23	24	25	26	27	28	29	30	32	33	34	35	36	37
6'8"	13	14	15	17	18	19	20	21	22	23	24	25	26	28	29	30	31	32	33	34	35	36
6'9"	13	14	15	16	17	18	19	20	21	23	24	25	26	27	28	29	30	31	32	33	34	35
6'10"	13	14	15	16	17	18	19	20	21	22	23	24	25	26	27	28	29	30	31	32	34	35

Severly Underweight: < 17.5   Optimal: 18.5 - 25   Overweight: 25.1 - 30   Obese: 30.1 - 40
Underweight: 17.5 - 18.4   Severely Obese: > 40.1

Table #1—BMI Index Table

Aerobic exercise: Brisk exercise that promotes the circulation of oxygen through the blood and is associated with an increased rate of breathing. Examples include running, swimming, and bicycling.

Obesity: It is a term to define how fat a person is.

It is defined in BMI as follows-Obesity is frequently subdivided into categories:

- Class 1: BMI of 30 to < 35
- Class 2: BMI of 35 to < 40
- Class 3: BMI of 40 or higher. Class 3 obesity is sometimes categorized as "extreme" or "severe" obesity.

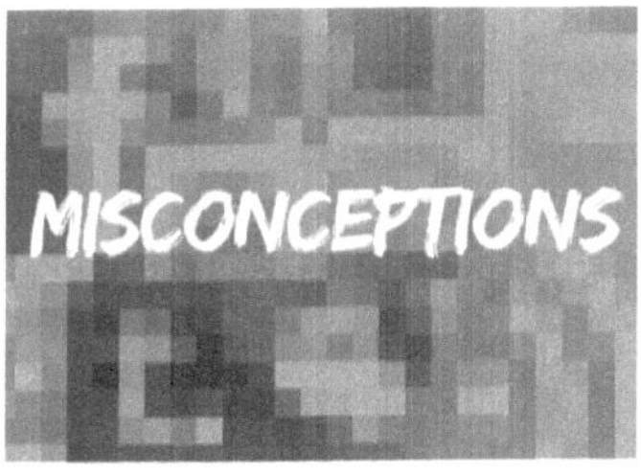

Misconceptions about Weight and Exercise

Common assumptions about how our weight and exercise affect our longevity are not always obvious.

For example, did you know that many medical studies have shown that if your overall weight is too low that can hurt your overall long term health and longevity? Here is what one study shows:

> *Researchers in Toronto, Canada found that people who are underweight have almost twice the risk of death as people who are obese. This finding came after a review of more than 50 previous studies. Some of the studies had followed patients for 5 or more years, focusing on relationships between body-mass index (or BMI, a measure doctors use to determine whether or not someone is at a healthy weight) and deaths from any cause. The studies also included deaths among newborns and still-born babies.*

And excessive weight may not affect us the way we think it does:

The best estimates of the association between body mass index (BMI) and mortality suggest that the mortality risk from excess body weight increases from a BMI of 25 but isn't substantial until BMI exceeds 32 or 35.

The previous statement is very interesting because if you look at Table 1 in the previous Chapter you will see that a BMI of 32 to 35 is well into the Obese Category.

This means the study is saying that the effects of overall health aren't a big factor until your BMI reaches the low thirties or more—into the Obese range.

Between 15% and 25% of the US population have BMIs in this range. While this is a significant proportion, it is nevertheless a minority. And the relationship between obesity and health appears to reverse in old age. **In old age, people who have low body weight are at higher risk of disability and mortality.** *But this reversal may be due to weight loss in old age due to disease.*

Indeed, body weight may not be a significant risk factor for mortality in itself. Instead it might simply be a surrogate marker for a particular lifestyle, or a particular diet, physical activity level, and genetic factors. If this were so, obese individuals would represent a heterogeneous group of people with high body weight for different reasons, some of which may not be strongly related to morbidity or mortality.

The previous statements from the study are really interesting because it shows that you cannot be an extremely obese person to avoid have long term health problems, but…

If you are in the "Lower" Obesity range your lifestyle may be more important that your weight for long term health.

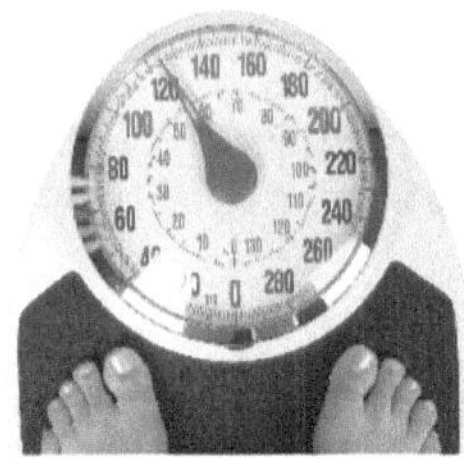

Studies on Weight

Being too thin can be as bad as being Obese. Another study shows:

Specific Reasons Why Being Underweight Is Unhealthy

Risk factors often found in people who are underweight include: malnourishment, drug or alcohol abuse, smoking, poverty, mental health issues (for example, people who are depressed or under severe stress may have diminished appetites and not eat enough), and even the belief that because one is thin, one does not need to go to the doctor for checkups. But the fact is that no matter what one's weight is, blood sugar levels and bad cholesterol levels can still be too high, and therefore unhealthy, even in an underweight individual.

A thin person might think that because they are underweight, they can eat unhealthy fast foods, avoid exercising and the like. But that is not the case.

In addition, people who are naturally very thin are often that way due to genetics. A 2011 study found that in thin people, fat may be stored deeper within the body, such as around vital organs like the heart and the liver. So, while a skinny person may not have the proverbial 'spare tire,' they may be carrying the fat that they do have in places that put them at higher risk for diabetes and even heart disease.

Being too thin can also work against a person's immunity. The body's immune cells need a variety of nutrients to take on invading germs; if a person doesn't eat very much, they are more likely to be missing out on key nutrients. This would decrease their ability to fight colds, allergies and different infections, including cancerous cells.

Anemia is another condition that many underweight people have; it is the result of nutritional deficiencies in iron, vitamin B-12 and folate. If you are underweight, it may be a good idea to have your doctor check for any nutritional deficiencies, and recommend foods that you need to eat more of.

And when it comes time to become a parent, an underweight woman or man is at a clear disadvantage. It is harder for an underweight woman to conceive, and it is also more difficult for her to sustain the pregnancy. One study found that underweight women were 72 percent more likely to have a miscarriage during the first trimester than women of a healthy weight. As for men, underweight men face a far greater risk — 22 times greater — of having sexual dysfunction, including erectile dysfunction, difficulty ejaculating and painful intercourse. The health of sperm may also be diminished in men who are underweight, according to previous studies.

Here is more information on how weight affects overall health from the Mayo Clinic:

Evidence for Weight and Longevity

I observed the obesity paradox in a published study I conducted while studying at the Mayo Clinic. We looked at 226 people who experienced a heart arrest in the community and were resuscitated.

What we found was that people that were slightly overweight (BMI from 25-30) had the highest 5-year survival at 78 percent. People who were underweight had a significantly lower survival at 67 percent, similar to people considered morbidly obese.

Our thoughts at that time with this study were similar to my colleague's now. We thought that thin cardiac arrest patients died more often because they were thin for a reason other than fitness. For example, they were thin because they had cancer, or were smokers, or had some other systemic disease.

Does the possibility of underweight people having other diseases explain the obesity paradox?

In a very nice study from the Mayo Clinic of 250, 152 patients from 40 different studies, the influence of weight on outcomes was further explored. The authors found that the lowest risk of all types of mortality as well as heart related mortality was in those people considered overweight (BMI from 25-30). In fact the risk of death was 12 percent lower than those people considered normal weight (BMI 20-24.9). The highest risk of mortality was in the underweight patients (BMI <20). Their risk was 37 percent higher than those people considered normal weight.

Even their risk of heart disease related mortality was higher (45 percent higher) than those that were normal weight.

It was not until people had a BMI >35 that there was a clear increased risk of heart disease related morality (80 percent increased risk) compared to normal weight people. This observation is a classic "U" shaped survival curve with the highest risks seen in those that were severely underweight or overweight, with the lowest part of the curve in those considered slightly overweight (BMI from 25-30).

These high mortality rates in the underweight people were recently evaluated in a long-term study looking at people over 30 years. In a study of

31,578 people from the Swiss National Cohort, the influence of body weight on long-term death risk was further explored. The authors defined being underweight as a BMI <19. Compared to being normal weight, those that were underweight had a much higher mortality risk (37 percent increased risk) regardless of smoking status. Furthermore, the authors could not find that the higher risk was associated by cancer, pulmonary or lung disease, or chronic heart disease.

These two studies suggest that diseases that make people thin are not fully responsible for the obesity paradox. Here is another article:

I went to the lead author of the large study from Mayo Clinic to get his opinion. Dr. Francisco Lopez-Jimenez is a world leader in cardiology with research interests in understanding the role of weight, body fat, and heart risks. When asked why the obesity paradox exists he said "Nobody knows the cause. All that we know is that incomplete adjustment (accounting for other disease processes) does not explain it". He offered potential explanations.

*1.	Obese people with coronary artery disease have a different disease process and often have risk factors for progression of disease that can be modified and as such respond better to treatments. For example, when we see an overweight person with high blood pressure, diabetes, and coronary artery disease we often talk about the central role* *of increasing activity and weight loss. Often when the weight goes down the blood pressure improves and the diabetes becomes more controllable. In this sense, the weight was related to risk factors (high blood pressure and diabetes). In underweight people with coronary artery disease and diabetes and high blood pressure the risk factors are often from genetic factors that may be less modifiable.*

2.   Underweight people often have less muscle. Obese people from the mere fact that they have to carry excess weight often develop more muscle in the legs and the thighs. Muscle mass itself is also a powerful predictor of mortality. Across multiple disease states and patient populations, people with more muscle mass do better and live longer.

3.   Fat may have a protective effect. Our bodies use fat for energy storage. In the process of fighting a disease we need energy. In people that have more energy stores that may have the ability to overcome a significant body insult from an acute or chronic disease. For example, an acute disease such as pneumonia or a chronic disease such as heart failure or emphysema.

Fitness is More Important than Being Thin:

In discussing this I don't want to promote weight gain. More importantly, I think there is more to daily health than weight and the pursuit of being underweight. In this regard, fitness is more than being thin and is more important than being thin.

Given the obesity paradox, I asked Dr. Lopez-Jimenez how he counsels patients regarding weight loss. He said "We emphasize that the paradox does not mean that an obese patient with coronary artery disease would not benefit from weight loss.

Nonsmokers have a better prognosis than smokers, but smokers who quit have a better prognosis than smokers who don't".

I believe this is very important advice. In the United States we are facing an obesity epidemic. A lot of this is driven by lifestyles that are less active and food sources that are calorie dense. Increasing activity needs to be an essential part of everybody's daily goals to improve their health. Healthy food choices can augment fitness and enhance muscle mass retention. Remember the mortality curves are "U" shaped, so those that were very obese (BMI >35) also had poor outcomes. Trying to maintain a healthy weight for your body frame still remains important and a fundament aspect the long-term health.

Maybe we should also conclude that the healthy ranges for BMI that the health profession uses might be skewed too much toward underweight levels. I.E. that BMI levels up to 30 are also healthy.

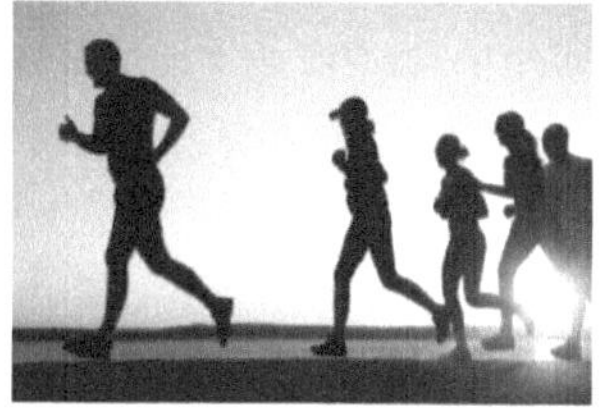

Studies on Exercise

Leisure-time physical activity is associated with longer life expectancy, even at relatively low levels of activity and regardless of body weight, according to a study by a team of researchers led by the National Cancer Institute (NCI), part of the National Institutes of Health. The study, which found that people who engaged in leisure-time physical activity had life expectancy gains of as much as 4.5 years, appeared Nov. 6, 2012, in PLoS Medicine Exit Disclaimer.

Effect of Body Weight & Physical Activity on Life Expectancy

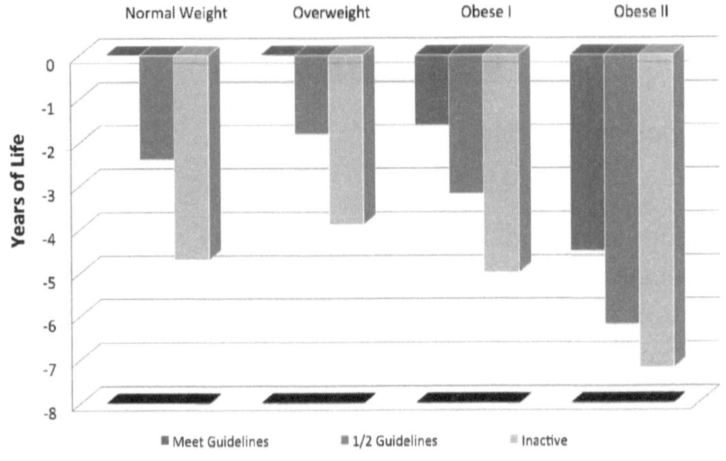

Chart #1

So the above chart shows the importance of exercise for all BMI levels.

You should still expect to have more health problems the higher your BMI, but exercise helps your overall health no matter what your weight.

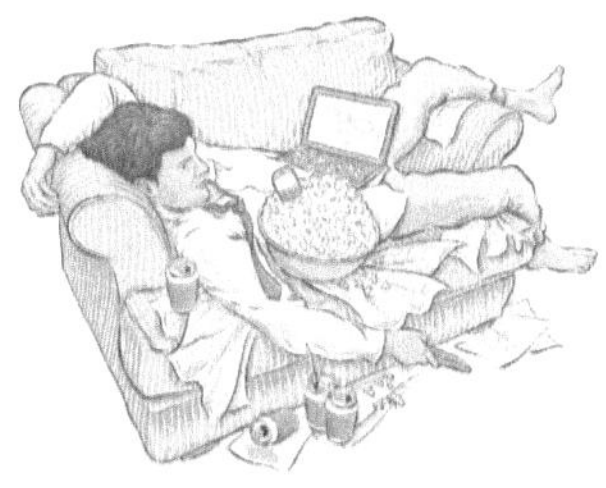

How Much Exercise Do You Need?

If you are a couch potato where you sit down at work all day, then come home to watch TV all evening and drink beer while doing so, then your health will obviously be bad.

So what is the minimum amount of exercise you need regularly to keep your body healthy?

Do you need to learn to run marathons, or will a simple regular workout suffice?

We are focusing on what is the minimum level of healthy exercise to maintain your long term health.

The Mayo Clinic has these exercise guidelines:

For most healthy adults, the Department of Health and Human Services recommends these exercise guidelines:

•   ***Aerobic activity*** *Get at least 150 minutes of moderate aerobic activity or 75 minutes of vigorous aerobic activity a week, or a combination of moderate and vigorous activity. The guidelines* *suggest that you spread out this exercise during the course of a week.*

*•   **Strength training.** Do strength training exercises for all major muscle groups at least two times a week. Aim to do a single set of each exercise, using a weight or resistance level heavy enough to tire your muscles after about 12 to 15 repetitions.*

Prevention.com has similar guidelines:

That dictum comes from the Centers for Disease Control and Prevention—and it's backed by plenty of studies, explains Lisa Cadmus-Bertram, PhD, an assistant professor of kinesiology at the University of Wisconsin–Madison. But the American College of Sports Medicine—a respected research group—refines the advice to say that if you go hard, your aerobic exercise can be just 75 minutes a week.

Of course, the ACSM experts also expect you to add strength training 2 to 3 days a week, and stretch on at least 2 days of every week.

So both sources say you need just 75 minutes or only 1 ¼ hours of aerobic exercise each week to stay healthy. This isn't really much to ask.

If you can put in 30 minutes of workouts just a few times per week you will meet this guideline.

Strength training is also considered important. You don't have to lift weights for strength training. There are other ways..

My preference is to do a thirty minute swim several times a week—It exercises all of my muscles.

Swimming is generally known as the most efficient overall aerobic exercise.

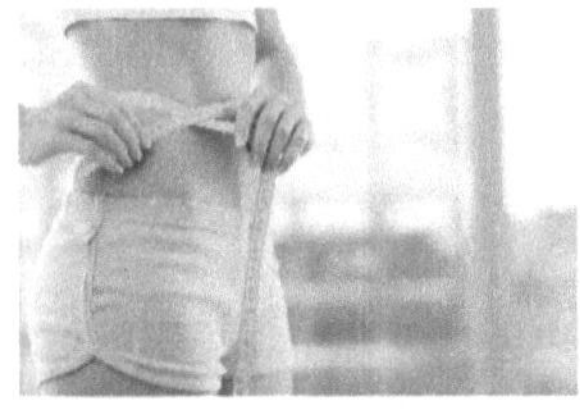

Advice on Weight loss

Like many of you readers I've had my own challenges over the years with keeping the weight off.

I remember that I used to eat everything and as much as I wanted… and my young metabolism burned everything off.

Then when I hit thirty years old my metabolism slowed significantly and I had to cut way down on what I was eating or I would gain lots of weight.

I've also done lots of diets and even went to weight loss centers. Unfortunately, I would lose significant weight under their programs then gain it all back within a couple of years.

The biggest thing I learned is that losing weight permanently is not about doing a diet, it's about living a healthy lifestyle.

My weight started to become under control when I switched from a diet heavy in meat and fats to being more vegetable oriented with chicken substituting for greasy and high calorie meets.

It also included a switch from sugary sodas to pure carbonated water or sometimes diet sodas.—but no more high sugar sodas.

I gave up sugary meals or desserts and kept myself from a fatty meal except maybe once a month. Generally sugar in foods and drinks is now cut out of my diet.

I also cut down drinking alcohol to only a little on some holidays. Maybe I'll have a glass of wine or two at a Christmas dinner, but that's all. Not having Alcohol in your system helps your weight loss and you avoid many other types of health problems.

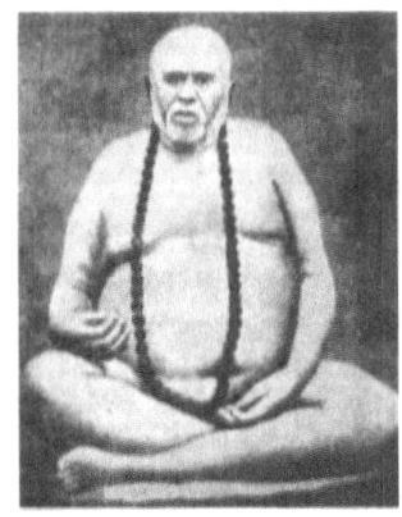

Mindfulness and Weight loss

I couldn't resist including a possible exception to the healthy weight rules.

Trialinga Swami was an Indian Yogi who supposedly lived to 280 and even possibly 300 years old.

His weight was supposedly over 300 pounds:

> He was reputed to have lived to be around 300 years, and was a larger-than-life figure, reportedly weighing over 300 pounds (140 kg), though he seldom ate. One account said that he could "read people's minds like books."

If he really did live that long and weighed that much then it was probably because his spiritual enlightenment gave him the effects of mindfulness which helped his body to retain its health.

Mindfulness practices have been shown in scientific studies to stabilize the Anterior Nervous System including organs and glands per the below picture:

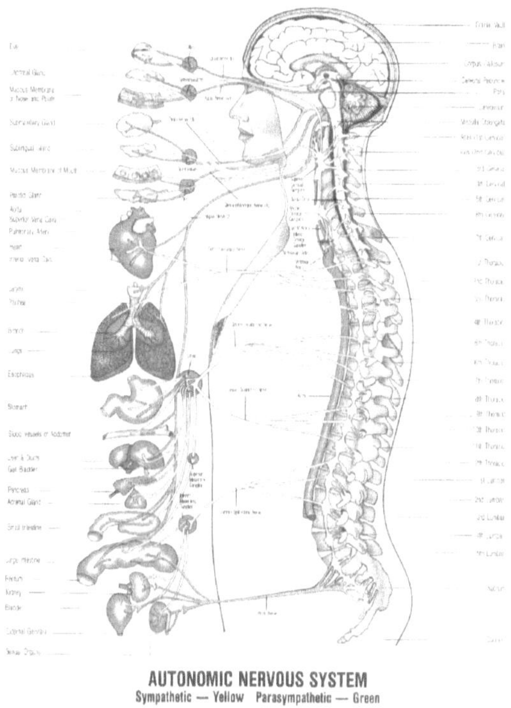

Figure 1

Mindfulness practices can also help control weight through reducing stress:

A quote from an article on Mindfulness:

Mindfulness is all about how one's mood, outlook, and ability to stay mindfully calm in the present moment can prevent unwanted weight gain and benefit overall health.

Being mindful includes the ability to control our reactions to ongoing, and often stressful, life events. Most would agree that we spend far too much time worrying about what has already happened in the past or what we fear may happen in the future.

While this response is an automatic reaction based on subconscious, limiting beliefs accumulated through life experience, many don't realize the huge impact that stress has on our health and even on our weight.

So mindfulness practices like meditation have a positive impact on stress and therefore often on our desires to eat.

Summary-Effects of Weight and Exercise On Longevity

This is just a short book on Weight and Exercise.

There are thousands of books out there on this subject and I didn't want to duplicate them.

My goal is to point out some key issues to keep in mind about how your weight and exercise influence your Longevity.

The key points are:

1) Your BMI can actually be up to 25 and the low end should be in the upper end of the healthy BMI range for the best effects on longevity from weight.
2) You only need 75 minutes of good aerobic exercise per week to maintain your long term health. I recommend double that just to be sure. Strength conditioning should be part of that time.
3) Successful weight control is about your lifestyle— not about a particular diet to lose weight.
4) Avoid processed Sugar as much as possible.
5) Mindfulness practices can reduce stress which can also have a major effect on your weight and overall health.

Summary

You know from the other books in this Longevity training series that I believe there are many other aspects important to Longevity besides the physical body.

But we can't neglect the importance of our bodies. It is obvious that without a healthy body we can't exist in this world, and there are lots of things you can do to have a healthy one.

The aspects of physical health we concentrated on in this book are not subjects you will find in your normal diet and exercise manual.

I hope you find this information useful in your quest to improve your longevity.